TEENS
AT RISK

Opposing Viewpoints®

Other Books of Related Interest

TEENS
AT RISK

Opposing Viewpoints®

Auriana Ojeda, *Book Editor*

Daniel Leone, *President*
Bonnie Szumski, *Publisher*
Scott Barbour, *Managing Editor*
Helen Cothran, *Senior Editor*

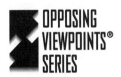

OPPOSING
VIEWPOINTS®
SERIES

GREENHAVEN
PRESS®

THOMSON
─────★─────
GALE

San Diego • Detroit • New York • San Francisco • Cleveland
New Haven, Conn. • Waterville, Maine • London • Munich

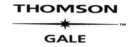

© 2003 by Greenhaven Press. Greenhaven Press is an imprint of The Gale Group, Inc., a division of Thomson Learning, Inc.

Greenhaven® and Thomson Learning™ are trademarks used herein under license.

For more information, contact
Greenhaven Press
27500 Drake Rd.
Farmington Hills, MI 48331-3535
Or you can visit our Internet site at http://www.gale.com

LIBRARY OF CONGRESS CATALOGING-IN-PUBLICATION DATA

Teens at risk : opposing viewpoints / Auriana Ojeda, book editor.
   p. cm. — (Opposing viewpoints series)
Includes bibliographical references and index.
ISBN 0-7377-1915-X (lib. bdg.) — ISBN 0-7377-1916-8 (pbk. : alk. paper)
   1. Teenagers with social disabilities—United States. 2. Problem youth—United States. 3. Juvenile delinquency—United States. 4. Teenage pregnancy—United States. 5. Teenagers—Substance use—United States. I. Ojeda, Auriana, 1977– .
II. Opposing viewpoints series (Unnumbered)
HV1431.T44 2003
362.74—dc21
                                               2003041768

Printed in the United States of America

"Congress shall make no law. . . abridging the freedom of speech, or of the press."

First Amendment to the U.S. Constitution

The basic foundation of our democracy is the First Amendment guarantee of freedom of expression. The Opposing Viewpoints Series is dedicated to the concept of this basic freedom and the idea that it is more important to practice it than to enshrine it.

Contents

Why Consider
Opposing Viewpoints?

*"The only way in which a human being can make some
approach to knowing the whole of a subject is by hearing
what can be said about it by persons of every variety of
opinion and studying all modes in which it can be looked
at by every character of mind. No wise man ever
acquired his wisdom in any mode but this."*

John Stuart Mill

In our media-intensive culture it is not difficult to find differing opinions. Thousands of newspapers and magazines
and dozens of radio and television talk shows resound with
differing points of view. The difficulty lies in deciding which
opinion to agree with and which "experts" seem the most
credible. The more inundated we become with differing
opinions and claims, the more essential it is to hone critical
reading and thinking skills to evaluate these ideas. Opposing
Viewpoints books address this problem directly by presenting stimulating debates that can be used to enhance and
teach these skills. The varied opinions contained in each
book examine many different aspects of a single issue. While
examining these conveniently edited opposing views, readers
can develop critical thinking skills such as the ability to
compare and contrast authors' credibility, facts, argumenta-
tion styles, use of persuasive techniques, and other stylistic
tools. In short, the Opposing Viewpoints Series is an ideal
way to attain the higher-level thinking and reading skills so
essential in a culture of diverse and contradictory opinions.

In addition to providing a tool for critical thinking, Opposing Viewpoints books challenge readers to question their
own strongly held opinions and assumptions. Most people
form their opinions on the basis of upbringing, peer pressure, and personal, cultural, or professional bias. By reading
carefully balanced opposing views, readers must directly
confront new ideas as well as the opinions of those with
whom they disagree. This is not to simplistically argue that

everyone who reads opposing views will—or should—change his or her opinion. Instead, the series enhances readers' understanding of their own views by encouraging confrontation with opposing ideas. Careful examination of others' views can lead to the readers' understanding of the logical inconsistencies in their own opinions, perspective on why they hold an opinion, and the consideration of the possibility that their opinion requires further evaluation.

Evaluating Other Opinions

To ensure that this type of examination occurs, Opposing Viewpoints books present all types of opinions. Prominent spokespeople on different sides of each issue as well as well-known professionals from many disciplines challenge the reader. An additional goal of the series is to provide a forum for other, less known, or even unpopular viewpoints. The opinion of an ordinary person who has had to make the decision to cut off life support from a terminally ill relative, for example, may be just as valuable and provide just as much insight as a medical ethicist's professional opinion. The editors have two additional purposes in including these less known views. One, the editors encourage readers to respect others' opinions—even when not enhanced by professional credibility. It is only by reading or listening to and objectively evaluating others' ideas that one can determine whether they are worthy of consideration. Two, the inclusion of such viewpoints encourages the important critical thinking skill of objectively evaluating an author's credentials and bias. This evaluation will illuminate an author's reasons for taking a particular stance on an issue and will aid in readers' evaluation of the author's ideas.

It is our hope that these books will give readers a deeper understanding of the issues debated and an appreciation of the complexity of even seemingly simple issues when good and honest people disagree. This awareness is particularly important in a democratic society such as ours in which people enter into public debate to determine the common good. Those with whom one disagrees should not be regarded as enemies but rather as people whose views deserve careful examination and may shed light on one's own.

Thomas Jefferson once said that "difference of opinion leads to inquiry, and inquiry to truth." Jefferson, a broadly educated man, argued that "if a nation expects to be ignorant and free . . . it expects what never was and never will be." As individuals and as a nation, it is imperative that we consider the opinions of others and examine them with skill and discernment. The Opposing Viewpoints Series is intended to help readers achieve this goal.

David L. Bender and Bruno Leone,
Founders

Greenhaven Press anthologies primarily consist of previously published material taken from a variety of sources, including periodicals, books, scholarly journals, newspapers, government documents, and position papers from private and public organizations. These original sources are often edited for length and to ensure their accessibility for a young adult audience. The anthology editors also change the original titles of these works in order to clearly present the main thesis of each viewpoint and to explicitly indicate the opinion presented in the viewpoint. These alterations are made in consideration of both the reading and comprehension levels of a young adult audience. Every effort is made to ensure that Greenhaven Press accurately reflects the original intent of the authors included in this anthology.

Introduction

"Living on the streets and on society's margins, runaways are the most vulnerable to the pestilences that kill America's teens: alcoholism, drugs, AIDS, homicide."
—John D. Hull

Many social critics argue that today's teenagers face significant risks that teens of other generations did not. In fact, a 1997 survey concluded that Americans are convinced that today's adolescents face a crisis. Experts contend that deteriorating family security, violence in schools, and alarming media images put teens at risk of not reaching their full potential. Teenagers who have difficulty coping with such tremendous stresses are more likely to engage in drug and alcohol abuse, sexual relationships that may result in unwanted pregnancies or sexually transmitted diseases, criminal acts, and suicide attempts. Many of these at-risk teens eventually find themselves living on the street after they run away from home or are thrown out or abandoned by their parents or guardians.

According to the National Runaway Switchboard (NRS), a national communication system for runaway and homeless youth, there are approximately 1.3 million people under the age of eighteen living on the streets in the United States. Some of these children are runaways, youth under the age of eighteen who are away from home for at least one night without the permission of their parents, guardians, or custodial authorities; others are throwaways, kids who were forced to leave home or were deserted by parents or guardians, many of whom are incarcerated, physically incapacitated, mentally ill, or addicted to drugs or alcohol. Although some runaways and throwaways are taken in by relatives or friends, many end up on the streets where risks to their well-being substantially increase. In fact, homeless youth are at greater risk of violence, sexual exploitation, and drug abuse than any other group of teenagers.

Poverty is the most ubiquitous problem facing street youths. Homeless children live in basements, abandoned buildings ("squats"), parks, train or bus stations, subways, and strangers' homes. They eat at youth shelters, forage for food in dumpsters, or steal food from restaurants and grocery stores. After they leave home, many teens try to find legitimate work, but most employers are reluctant to hire them because of their youth. Most of them struggle to live on handouts but quickly realize that they cannot survive on charity. As stated by the NRS, "They may start by panhandling for change, but eventually a [street youth] will most likely turn to illegal means to survive; many will become involved in prostitution, pornography, drugs, stealing, and other crimes." Many homeless teens engage in "survival sex," exchanging sexual favors for food, a place to stay, protection, or drugs.

A 2001 study found that approximately 70 percent of street youth engage in prostitution to meet their everyday needs for food, shelter, or drugs. According to the NRS, about 49 percent of teenage prostitutes are girls, and 51 percent are boys. Experts contend that pimps and other street predators target homeless youths because teens who have recently left home are particularly vulnerable and desperate for money. Pimps earn a street youth's trust by giving him or her intense attention and affection for a short period of time, and by making false claims that prostitution is a fun and easy way to make a lot of money. However, young prostitutes quickly learn that hustling is a dangerous activity. Young prostitutes risk rape, assault, and murder at the hands of johns. In addition, they are usually extremely dependent on their pimps, who frequently physically abuse them, force them to turn as many tricks as possible, and confiscate the money they make. Moreover, teenage prostitutes are at increased risk of unplanned pregnancy and contracting HIV and other sexually transmitted diseases. The NRS reports that HIV rates are two to ten times higher among street youth than among other adolescents.

In light of the incredible risks associated with living on the street, it is natural to wonder how so many teens become homeless. The vast majority—approximately 65 percent—of homeless youth have run away from home. Some children run away because of typical rebellion or everyday family conflict, but experts agree that most youth run away to escape physical, sexual, or emotional abuse at home. According to Kevin Jackson, street outreach manager at the Our Town Family Center in Tucson, Arizona, "Something has gone wrong. [Kids are unlikely to leave a good home] unless they have some sort of emotional or psychological issues that preclude them from being attached to that family." Numerous studies support Jackson's theory. Two 1997 studies by the U.S. Department of Health and Human Services (HHS) found that 46 percent of runaway and homeless youth reported being physically abused, 17 percent reported being sexually exploited, and 38 percent reported being emotionally abused at home. In a survey published by the National Association of Social Workers (NASW), 66 percent of runaway and homeless youth reported having an alcoholic parent, and 25 percent reported having a parent who abused drugs. Another study found that 40 percent of girls and 30 percent of boys who engaged in prostitution had been sexually abused at home.

Runaways voluntarily leave home, but a significant portion of street youth are "throwaways," kids who were forced to leave their parents' house or were abandoned by their parents or guardians. Many teens are thrown out of their homes because their parents find out that they are gay, are having sex, are pregnant, or are on drugs, or because they fail to follow their parents' rules. A study by HHS determined that throwaways account for 12 to 36 percent of all homeless youth. These children are sometimes more susceptible to the risks of street life than are other homeless youth because, unlike most runaways, throwaways cannot return home. As a consequence, many throwaways feel rejected by their families and seek comfort in risky behaviors such as drug use and prostitution. As stated by writer Elizabeth Barfield, "[Throwaways], some not even teenagers yet, do not have a choice; there is no place for them. . . . [T]hey cannot call home, ask forgiveness, and be sent a bus ticket. There is no home to call."

While many homeless youth are unable to go home, there are a variety of government programs and private organizations that offer services to children living on the street. Since 1974, Congress has funded three grant programs under the Runaway and Homeless Youth Act: Basic Center Training,

Transitional Living, and Street Outreach. The Basic Center Training program provides financial assistance to programs that address the immediate needs of homeless youth, such as food, clothing, shelter, and medical attention. These programs set up emergency shelters and soup kitchens, and strive to reunite young people with their families when possible. The Transitional Living program supports agencies that provide longer-term residential services to homeless youth between the ages of sixteen and twenty-one for up to eighteen months. Living accommodations include host family homes, group homes, or "supervised apartments"—apartment buildings that are owned by the agency. The Street Outreach program provides grants to private, nonprofit organizations that try to pass information about safe, healthy living to youth living on the street. They also offer homeless youth medical treatment, counseling, and other resources and try to bring some street children into shelters for more in-depth assistance. Homeless youth can also contact numerous nongovernmental help services and hotlines.

Despite the resources available to runaways and throwaways, the risks that homeless youth face continue to rise because the number of children living on the street increases every year. Unfortunately, homelessness is only one of many factors that put young people at risk. Other factors include teen sex and pregnancy, crime, drug and alcohol abuse, and tobacco use. *Teens at Risk: Opposing Viewpoints* examines how society can deal with homeless and other at-risk youth in the following chapters: What Factors Put Teens at Risk? How Can the Adverse Consequences of Teenage Sex and Pregnancy Be Reduced? How Can Society Deal with Teenage Crime and Violence? How Can Teen Substance Abuse Be Reduced? In these chapters, authors assess the risks that today's teens face and present potential solutions to their problems.

What Factors Put Teens at Risk?

Chapter Preface

Experts contend that suicide rates are a major indicator of whether teens are at risk. Recent studies have found an alarming increase in teen suicides over the last few decades. In 1960 the suicide rate among fifteen- to nineteen-year-olds was 3.6 per one hundred thousand. By 1990, 11.1 out of every one hundred thousand teenagers ages fifteen and older committed suicide, according to the U.S. Centers for Disease Control and Prevention (CDC). Surgeon General David Satcher has called teen suicide "the nation's hidden epidemic."

A 1997 Youth Risk Behavior Survey found that for every teenager who commits suicide, one hundred more will attempt it. Every year one in thirteen high school students attempts suicide, and half of all high school students claim that they have "seriously considered" killing themselves by the time they graduate, the study found. Thus, an estimated seven hundred thousand American teenagers try to kill themselves every year, and millions say that they have contemplated doing so.

Teenage girls attempt suicide three times more often than boys do, but boys are four times more likely to be successful. Experts contend that boys succeed more often than girls because boys choose more lethal means of suicide—such as firearms and hanging—than do girls, who favor less violent methods, such as overdosing on pills. Girls attempt suicide more often than boys, according to experts, because attempting suicide is an effort to communicate their despair. Boys, on the other hand, tend to keep their emotions hidden. As stated by Harvard psychiatry professor William Pollack, "Girls cry out for help, while boys are taught to be tough and never to act like a 'girl'. [As a result,] boys are so ashamed of their feelings they figure they'd be better off dead [than communicate their desperation]."

Sociologists and mental-health experts associate a variety of physiological, cultural, and psychological factors with the recent increase in teen suicide. Such factors include poor impulse control due to raging hormones; a deluge of violent images on television, in movies, and in video games; increased availability of handguns; and increases in mental-health

17

problems such as depression. Professionals also maintain that teenagers are natural risk-takers who may not fully comprehend the finality of their actions. Teenagers often see suicide as the end of their problems, not their lives. According to Tom Simon, a suicide researcher at the CDC, "The developmental stage of adolescence is consistent with not thinking of the long- or short-term consequences of behavior."

In addition to adolescent impulsivity, many health professionals point to a decline of the traditional family unit as a major cause of teenage suicide. Statistics reveal that the teenage suicide rate began its ascent just as the divorce rate started to climb in the 1970s. Half of U.S. marriages now end in divorce, compared with 28 percent in the 1960s; 70 percent of minors who try to kill themselves have parents who are divorced. Experts contend that the disintegration of the family unit makes children more vulnerable because they lose a solid familial support system. These children are more likely to engage in self-destructive behaviors than a child from an intact family.

Suicide is just one behavior that threatens teens' lives. The authors in the following chapter debate other factors that put teens at risk.

> "Up to 15% of 16- to 19-year-olds are at
> risk of never reaching their potential and
> simply becoming lost in society."

A Variety of Factors Put Teens at Risk

Gene Stephens

In the following viewpoint, Gene Stephens argues that the number of at-risk teens is growing. He contends that a combination of social ills—such as teenage pregnancy, child abuse, and poor health care—and individual problems—such as truancy, drug abuse, and feelings of hopelessness—put today's teens at risk. He suggests that implementing community-based youth programs can lead troubled youth in a positive direction. Stephens is a professor of criminal justice at the University of South Carolina.

As you read, consider the following questions:
1. Why does James Fox believe that murders by juveniles will skyrocket in the first decade of the twenty-first century?
2. According to Stephens, what are the consequences of inadequate health care?
3. What examples does the author give of "community-oriented proactive policing programs"?

Gene Stephens, "Youth at Risk: Saving the World's Most Precious Resource," *Futurist*, vol. 31, March/April 1997, p. 31. Copyright © 1997 by World Future Society. Reproduced by permission.

Growing numbers of children are being neglected, abused, and ignored. Without change, the dark specter of generational warfare could become all too real.

After two decades of study, however, I conclude that we can stop this negative trend and do a better job of nourishing this most important resource. To do otherwise would surely be a violation of our obligation to future generations.

Child-care advocates claim that up to 15% of 16- to 19-year-olds are at risk of never reaching their potential and simply becoming lost in society. Others would add to this category children of any age if they are at risk of not becoming self-supporting adults, headed for a life in institutions for delinquency, crime, mental illness, addiction, and dependency. We could also describe as "at risk" those teens and preteens who take on child rearing themselves and drop out of school.

Saving the Children

The task of saving these children has become increasingly formidable. Compounding the problem are the expanding gap between the rich and poor, the increasing number of single-parent households, the rise of homes where both parents work, the growing gun culture, and the recent increase in negative attitudes about children, such as courts that treat younger and younger children as adult criminals.

As a result, children lose hope for the future. They turn to peers for attention; they turn to guns for protection, security and status; and they turn to sex and drugs for comfort and relief of boredom. The gang too often becomes their "family"—the only place where they receive attention and approval.

Criminologist James Fox of Northeastern University predicts that the murders committed by teenagers (4,000 in the United States in 1995) will skyrocket as the 39 million children now under age 10 swell the ranks of teenagers by 20% in the first decade of the twenty-first century. The result could be a juvenile crime wave such as the United States has never seen.

Yet, such a catastrophe is not inevitable. There are some signs of hope: a slightly decreased birth rate among teenagers in the mid-1990s, a rising bipartisan concern about "saving the children," burgeoning community-based experiments for meeting the needs of youth, and a movement to regard poor prenatal care, poor parenting skills, child abuse, and child neglect as public-health problems.

Beyond this, a striking change in the rearing of children in many families has been observed. Countering the trend toward ignoring or even abusing children is a trend toward cherishing and nurturing them. Thousands or even millions of young parents are taking turns working while the other stays at home and makes child care almost a full-time vocation. There is an unrecognized renaissance in parenting progressing quietly in neighborhoods across the nation and possibly the world.

Of course, having youth at risk is not a problem unique to the United States. Wars, social upheaval, rapidly changing economic systems, political instability, and cultural animosity have placed millions of children at risk around the world. Children die of starvation while others wander aimlessly in search of home and family. . . .

Teenage Pregnancy

Many child advocates see teenage pregnancy as the main problem. Children having children puts both generations at risk and often leads to poverty, poor health care, truancy, and underemployment. The dimensions of the issue—as reported by the National Commission on Children, the United States Census Bureau, and others—are staggering:

- Every year, one in 10 teenage females becomes pregnant—more than 3,000 a day.
- One of four teenage mothers will have a second child within one year of her first child's birth.
- Most teenage mothers are single and receive no support from the father.
- Eight of 10 teenage mothers do not finish high school.

About one-fourth of the families in America are headed by a single parent—usually the mother. In the Hispanic community, it is one-third; among black families, it is one-half. Most of the children in these families were born to teenagers.

According to the Centers for Disease Control (CDC), 85% of all children exhibiting behavioral disorders came from fatherless homes. Other statistical findings indicate that children from fatherless homes are: 32 times more likely to run away; nine times more likely to drop out of high school; 14 times more likely to commit rape; 10 times more likely to be substance abusers; and 20 times more likely to end up in prison.

Poverty

Whereas 75% of single-female-headed households are in poverty at least some of the time, and 33% are chronically poor, poverty is also endemic to a majority of young households. Already, one in three children under 6 lives below the poverty line.

About half of the homeless are families with children. A million divorces each year create new female-headed households below the poverty line.

Poor Health Care

CDC and other agencies have found that at least 25 million children in the United States have no health care. This means that they are taken to the hospital emergency room or to nonprofessionals for health problems. Without change in health provider arrangements, half of the nation's children could [soon] be without health care. . . . Already, most unwed mothers receive no prenatal care.

Lack of health care too often equals stunted ability to learn, life-altering health problems, lowered ability to cope in a free-market system, and, as a result, greater likelihood of drug abuse, delinquency, and crime.

Child Abuse

There is substantial evidence of child abuse or neglect in the background of every known serial killer. In most cases, the abuse was physically or sexually severe.

Beyond blatant abuse, neglect itself—ignoring the child's physical and emotional needs—is a form of abuse that scars the child as much or more than beatings.

Child abuse and neglect are often called the "silent epidemic" in the United States. Alleged abuse more than quadrupled between the mid-1970s and the mid-1990s to more than

3 million cases a year reported (and 1 million substantiated]

A Gallup Poll reported that physical abuse cases were 10 times greater than reported rates, and sexual abuse was 10 times greater.

Increase in Risk-Taking Behaviors

The Carnegie Council [ethics and education research organization] reported that in a recent graduating high school class, 92% had consumed alcohol, and of those, 56% had begun in the sixth through ninth grades, while 36% had begun in the tenth through twelfth grades. These numbers do not include those who had dropped out of school, and who were even more likely to use alcohol. Problem behaviors are also interrelated. For example, young people who drink often experiment with illegal drugs. They may smoke and engage in unprotected sex. These same adolescents are more prone to school failure.

More teenagers are becoming sexually active before the age of 16, and girls are becoming pregnant at a greater rate and dropping out of school early. Young mothers are usually economically disadvantaged, have limited opportunities, and their pregnancies lead disproportionately to the birth of low-weight babies who are vulnerable to many poor outcomes. It has been estimated that one-fourth of all sexually active adolescents will become infected with a sexually transmitted disease before graduating from high school, AIDS being the greatest concern.

With the increase in risk-taking behaviors and substance abuse, motor vehicle deaths are also increasing. This is true particularly among those aged 10 to 14 years. This results from association with older adolescents who have been drinking. For this same age group, between 1980 and 1985 the suicide rate doubled. Seriously delinquent activities are peaking now at the age of 15, and of the 28 million boys and girls aged 10 to 17 in the U.S., 14 million are at moderate or high risk due to substance use and other deleterious behaviors. The cost of these behaviors to society is several billion dollars.

Don Martin and Maggie Martin, *Adolescence*, Winter 2000.

The U.S. Department of Justice reports that abused or neglected children are 40% more likely to be arrested as juvenile delinquents and adult criminals; three times as likely to use drugs and alcohol, get into fights, and deliberately damage property; and four times as likely to steal and be arrested. It is also reported that one in eight neglected children was later arrested for a violent offense.

Chronic Truancy and School Dropout

On the average school day, as many as 15% of junior and senior high school students are not in school. For too many, this is a pattern that leads to dropout.

Truants represent a large portion of those arrested for daytime break-ins and thefts, and dropouts are over-represented in jails and prisons.

The Census Bureau reports that earnings of students without a high school diploma average far below the poverty line.

Alcohol and Drug Abuse

Polls of youth indicate that 9 out of 10 teenagers drink alcohol to some extent by the time they finish high school, and a majority have used illegal drugs. A study of 1,200 school dropouts in California found their weekly alcohol-use rates were twice as high as in-school counterparts, and their use of hard drugs was two to five times as high. Dropout drug users were much more likely to be involved in violent and criminal activities. One-third said they had sold drugs in the past year, and twice as many dropouts as in-school students said they belonged to a gang.

Lack of Faith in Tomorrow

The Gallup Poll reported that 70% of 16- to 24-year-olds believe that the world was a better place when their parents were their age, and 56% said it will be worse for their own children. A joint *Washington Post*, Kaiser, and Harvard survey reported that the belief that "most people can be trusted" fell from 54% to 35%, and trust in government dropped from 76% to 25% over a three-decade period ending in 1995. At-risk youth, in particular, say they "live for today" and see no hope for their future.

Crime and Homicide

In 1996, the Justice Department reported that the juvenile homicide rate had almost doubled in over a decade, and blacks and males were by far the most likely to be killed.

The major correlating factor was an increase in the use of firearms. Guns were also found to be the single factor that could account for tripling the number of juvenile homicide offenders over the decade. Justice predicts another doubling of crime by juveniles by 2010 if current trends continue.

Tragically, most victims of juvenile violence are other juveniles, often children who are not even involved in the dispute. . . .

A Plan

The plan that follows represents a consensus from groups to whom I've given the same assignment over the past decade: "Develop a program to turn your community's youth into productive, happy, law-abiding adults." These groups have included students from high school to graduate school, practitioners from police to social service workers, and community leaders, all participating in brainstorming and planning sessions to alleviate the youth-at-risk problem.

Here is a comprehensive plan based on my 10-plus years' experience with these exercises.

1. Commit to positive reinforcement through community and school-based parenting classes (mandatory in schools), ongoing media campaigns, positive attention, and recognition in all schools (preschool through high school) and community-based programs.
2. Promote nonviolent conflict resolution among peers through mandatory educational programs for students, parents, teachers, counselors, administrators, media, and community campaigns.
3. Encourage mentoring for all children. Civic, business, and community campaigns should recruit and train mentors, matching them by needs and temperament. Programs such as Big Brothers and Big Sisters should be expanded.
4. Establish community-school partnerships to offer before- and after-school tutoring. Enlist youth to perform services to the community to enhance their stake in society.
5. Develop community-oriented proactive policing pro-

grams that begin with a philosophy of prevention. Examples of prevention programs include midnight basketball leagues, police-youth athletic leagues, neighborhood housing project substations, and foot patrols. These all involve partnerships of police, parents, church, business, civic, and community organizations.

6. Initiate ethical and cultural awareness programs that build on partnerships among family, church, school, media, civic, business, and other community groups. These programs would emphasize finding common ground on basic values, such as respect, responsibility, and restraint.

7. Design youth opportunity programs to provide all children the chance to reach their potential, regardless of circumstances. Such programs could be run through school, business, and community partnerships that provide in-school jobs and child care, career counseling and training, opportunity scholarships, and recognition for achievement.

8. Set up peer counseling hotlines to help youth help each other through the trying times of adolescence.

To this basic plan we may also consider in the future adding more dramatic (though often controversial) measures, such as birth-control implants, health monitoring and treatment implants, behavioral control implants in extreme cases, computer-assisted brain implants, and educational implants. But these measures should only be considered after reaching consensus concerning ethical issues.

In addition, we must focus on justice where delinquency and crime occur. Youth offenders must recognize the consequences of their actions on the victim, the victim's family, and the community. The harm must be ameliorated and restored through mediation and arbitration, restitution, service to the victim and community, reclamation, and reconciliation.

Final Thoughts

Every community can develop programs guided by this model. But all plans must adopt certain guiding principles that permeate the approach.

Children want attention above everything. Thus, giving

attention reinforces behavior and denying attention extinguishes behavior. Both praise and punishment are attention, and both will reinforce behavior that gets that attention.

It is important to instill optimism and faith in the future in all children, as they are the key to success. The very nature of adolescence is to challenge authority, but most children drift through this troubled period and become law-abiding adults unless they become labeled as delinquents, criminals, or losers.

Surely we can see the need to reach out and lend a hand to the world's most precious resource.

> *"The latest . . . statistics show the hazards of being a . . . teen at record lows."*

Teens Are Not at Risk

Mike Males

University of Santa Cruz sociology professor Mike Males challenges the argument that teenagers are at risk. In fact, he contends, today's teens produce higher academic achievement scores, more college graduates, fewer teenage pregnancies, and less drug addiction than their counterparts did twenty years ago. Males argues that today's teens are remarkably successful given the troubled world they inherited from their parents.

As you read, consider the following questions:
1. What positive social habits do adults no longer associate with youth, according to the author?
2. As described by Males, what are two examples of middle-age and elder selfishness?
3. What does the author contend explains healthier youth behavior?

Mike Males, "The True 'Great Generation,'" *Los Angeles Times*, August 26, 2001, p. M-1. Copyright © 2001 by Los Angeles Times Syndicate. Reproduced by permission.

Check out your favorite bookstore's newer "parenting" and "adolescence" arrivals, and you will find many of their authors decrying the degeneration of modern youth. Today's teens are lonely, troubled, depressed and confused, say psychologists William S. Pollack and Mary Bray Pipher. "Twice as many kids . . . are seriously troubled" and exalt "dark images," worries psychologist James Garbarino. Today's teenage girls engage "in far riskier health behavior in greater numbers than any prior generation," claims leftist media critic Jean Kilbourne. Youths perpetrate "our most troubling social problems," asserts rightist philosopher Kay S. Hymowitz. "Substance abuse has become epidemic. . . . 5,000 adolescents take their lives every year and the increase in adult crimes (theft, robbery, murder) committed by children [are] frightful evidence of . . . [a] new morbidity," says psychologist David Elkind.

Straight-Line Thinking

However, the latest statistics show that youth crime and drug and alcohol abuse, among other social ills, are plunging. Mindful of these, generational historians Neil Howe and William Strauss argue, in *Millennials Rising: The Next Great Generation*, that the new Millennials (youngsters born after 1981) "manifest a wide array of positive social habits that older Americans no longer associate with youth: teamwork, achievement, modesty and good conduct." Commentators who assume that Millennials will continue the "selfishness in personal manner . . . risk-taking with sex and drugs [and] crime, violence and social decay" of grungy-gangsta Generation X (born 1961–1981) commit fallacious "straight-line thinking," the authors contend.

What both the optimistic Howe and Strauss and the negativist others suggest is that stern adult authority produces model kids, while freedom yields brats. While the negativists call for renewed grown-up authority to "rescue," "revive" and "save" the wayward young, Howe and Strauss argue that adult crackdowns on youths in the 1990s have already nullified the effects of 30 years of permissiveness to forge disciplined, "no-nonsense kids."

But this homily wilts in the face of reality. The permissively raised, universally deplored Generation X (especially California's version) is the true "great generation," for it has braved a hostile social climate to reverse the abysmal trends of their baby-boomer predecessors.

Boomers' youthful difficulties are understandable legacies of the politically and morally turbulent 1960s. But three decades of adult arrogance, selfishness and puritanical hypocrisy since then are not. Sixties boomers pushed peace, civil rights and noble ideals; in the 1990s, they presided over a draconian war on drugs, resegregation and me-first politics. Boomers owe their record affluence to free quality education and opportunities paid for by their elders. But when it came their turn to pay the bills, they slashed their taxes and imposed sacrifices on youth. Ceaseless in their praise of "family values," boomers constitute America's most family-destroying adults ever. Modern authorities who slander teenagers as bearers of drugs, crime and egocentrism are really describing boomers.

Selfish Older Generations

Middle-age and elder selfishness has taken an appalling toll. California's once-exemplary public schools, universities and youth services deteriorated because of layoffs and overcrowding after older voters awarded themselves nearly 60% in tax cuts, beginning with Proposition 13 in 1978. The state's per-pupil funding fell from fifth nationally to 37th in 1998. University tuition rocketed 600% in real dollars. Student debts soared from near zero in the 1960s to $4 billion in the 1990s. The percentage of impoverished youth doubled as industries slashed jobs and young-family income fell 20%. Twice as many Gen-Xer children grew up in fractured non-families, as drug abuse, arrest and imprisonment tripled among their parents, whose average marriage lasted 80 months.

Given such a harsh initiation, Gen-Xers should have been disastrously messed up. Not so. California's detailed, long-term statistics document the amazing improvements Gen-Xers have brought. As the state's teenage population rose by half a million from the 1970s to the 1990s, teenage drug-abuse deaths plummeted from 200 to 30 a year; felony arrests dropped 50%; property crime plunged 60%; drunken-driving fatalities fell from 300 to fewer than 100 annually; cigarette smoking declined 40%; suicidal deaths decreased from 600 to fewer than 300 annually; pregnancy dropped 20%; and sexually transmitted diseases declined by half. Even amid crowded, underfunded schools, Gen-Xers' 1998 Scholastic Aptitude Test scores were, on average, 15 points above boomers' 1975 nadir.

Boomers laud themselves as socially conscious, but studies show that Gen-Xers are the real, in-the-trenches community volunteers. Far from the depressed, alienated misfits today's psychologist-authors bemoan, surveys consistently find 80% to 90% of Gen-Xers self-confident and optimistic.

Perceptions of Perfection

In a 1997 *U.S. News & World Report* poll, Americans picked the 1950s as their favorite decade in the century for being an adolescent. Two in 5 Americans say they would have liked to have been a teen then, a time when many more families were intact, and violent crime was much rarer than today. But life was often hard for adolescents in the 1950s, too. Black students in the South endured apartheid-like oppression, and nationwide, more than two thirds of black students dropped out of high school. Millions of girls around the country felt that it was inappropriate or unnecessary to go on to college.

Drinking by teens was also every bit as bad as it is today, and children were much more likely to live in poverty and die prematurely. Adolescents couldn't contract AIDS, but they could get polio—in 1952, almost 60,000 children were stricken with the disease. Older male teens had to join the military, and often risked their lives in Korea and later, in the 60s, in Vietnam—as opposed to enlisting chiefly to receive training or scholarship aid, as youth do today. More than 11,000 of the names on the Vietnam Veterans Memorial wall are those of 18- and 19-year-olds.

David Whitman, *U.S. News & World Report*, May 5, 1997.

The few bad Gen-Xer trends—notably, the early-1990s surge in teen births, street violence and murder—principally afflicted youth suffering from high unemployment and poverty. It was not permissive parenting, but aging boomers' demand for crack cocaine and heroin that touched off the drug-supply warfare and gang violence in the inner cities. In the late 1990s, crime rates among the state's poorest black and Latino youths dropped to levels below those of the 1970s. Imprisonment of California's young black men fell 35% during the 1990s, while drug abuse and imprisonment among white and black men over age 30 soared, statistics that challenge the familiar nostrum that older men should "rescue" young inner-city males. Despite claims of rising suicide, a black teen today is only one-third as likely to take his own life as his 1970 counterpart.

Trends among California's white kids, purportedly the most permissively indulged, show that Gen-Xer improvements would have been more spectacular had their elders not imposed the poverty and disinvestment that endangered poorer youth. White teens comprise California's fastest-declining criminal population. Every year in the 1970s, about 55,000 white youth were arrested for felonies and 80 were charged with murder. By contrast, the respective 1990s statistics are 25,000 felonies and 50 murders a year.

"Toxic" Teen Culture

In the 1990s, psychologists warned that teen culture had turned "toxic," yet white teens' safety improved amazingly: Rates of suicide, gun death and murder fell 40%; drug-related deaths dropped 45%; and all deaths as a result of violence plunged 50%. By the mid-1990s, California Gen-Xers had erased the perils that boomers had brought at every age level. A University of California, Los Angeles, (UCLA) survey comparing 1992 freshman girls with their 1969 counterparts said it all: The former boasted three times the varsity sports letters, and only one-seventh as many took sedatives.

Now, the Millennial teens, despite rare but terrible exceptions such as school shootings, are extending the Gen-Xers' improvements. The latest—1999—statistics show the hazards of being a California teen at record lows: suicide, lowest level since 1959; homicide, lowest since 1967; violent and other felony crime, lowest since 1967; drug deaths, a bit higher than Gen-Xers' but still 80% below boomers' rates; violent death, lowest ever; and birth rates, lowest since 1940.

What caused this unexpectedly healthier youth behavior? Howe and Strauss' answer, mostly based on anecdotal evidence, credits curfews, school uniforms, a "zero tolerance" drug policy, curriculum standards and strict parenting. Malarkey! The two decades of impressive Gen-Xer improvements long predated the current get-tough fervor, and accumulating research shows that curfews, zero tolerance and other responses to youth troubles are feckless.

A more positive—and revealing—answer may be that Gen-Xers compensated for their boomer parents' disarray by assuming more adult responsibilities at younger ages and refusing to emulate their elders' excesses. Contrary to their detractors, Gen-Xer teens proved admirably competent in handling adult freedoms and duties. The most worrisome question is whether boomers, whose political power is peaking, will reverse or exacerbate their record as the generation that wrecked California's once-rich promise to its young.

> "*Teenagers today are more likely to die of gunshot wounds than of all natural causes combined.*"

A Violent Society Puts Teens at Risk

Peggy O'Mara

In the following viewpoint, Peggy O'Mara contends that Americans' obsession with guns combined with high rates of child abuse and neglect creates violent, angry teenagers. Moreover, according to O'Mara, an increasingly powerful and centralized media pushes materialism and violence on the nation's youth. She maintains that the best way to reduce the number of at-risk teens is for parents to spend more time with their teenagers and for small, committed groups to challenge the commercial interests that control the media. O'Mara is the publisher of *Mothering* magazine, a journal dedicated to celebrating parenthood and family.

As you read, consider the following questions:

1. According to O'Mara, what does the American Academy of Pediatrics (AAP) suggest that pediatricians do to protect children?
2. What effect does bullying have on teenagers, according to the author?
3. How did the British government react to a 1995 school shooting in Scotland, as described by the author?

In the days and weeks following the Columbine [school] shootings in Colorado in April 1999, everyone walked around in a daze. Some watched everything on TV. Others didn't talk about it. We were all in shock. No one knew what to think.

I had written the editorial "Children Who Kill" after the Oregon shootings [in May 1998, when a fifteen-year-old boy shot and killed two classmates at school, and then went home and shot his parents] and thought I had some ideas about the roots of violence, but the Columbine shootings do not lend themselves to easy answers. We must, however, find the answers and make Columbine a turning point in the history of violence in US society.

Are We a Violent Society?

In order to understand Columbine, I had to first answer the question of whether or not we are, in fact, a violent society. While this is a common belief, few of us know how frequent shootings like the Columbine incident really are and what the incidence of violence actually is in the US.

Following a two-year analysis of violence and children, the American Academy of Pediatrics (AAP) issued a new policy in January 1999 recommending preventative measures to curtail the spread of what it calls an epidemic. This is the first time a US medical association has acknowledged that violence is a health issue, not only a criminal justice issue.

"Violence has become increasingly prominent . . . in the United States, which has the highest youth homicide and suicide rates among 26 wealthiest nations in the world and one of the highest rates of homicide worldwide," the AAP says. While there is a general decline in US homicides nationwide, violence and violent injuries among children have not decreased.

Homicide and suicide have become the second and third leading causes of death of all teenagers, and the leading cause of death among black youths. Homicide rates for males 15 to 19 years of age increased 113 percent between 1985 and 1995. Teenagers today are more likely to die of gunshot wounds than of all natural causes combined.

According to the AAP, violent injury and death result far

more often from altercations between family members and acquaintances than from robberies or other criminal activity.

Risk Factors for Violence

To help the nation's pediatricians assess and screen patients, the new AAP policy identifies risk factors such as substance abuse problems, history of mental illness, family stresses that could lead to violence, and exposure to violence at home and in the media.

As part of the efforts to deter violence and violence-related injuries, the AAP suggests that pediatricians embark on a variety of advocacy efforts on behalf of children. These include support for quality, affordable child care, reduced corporal punishment, and reduced availability or elimination of handguns.

To prevent violence before it starts, the AAP also addresses research on early brain development and offers pediatricians guidance on age-appropriate development for children from birth through late adolescence.

What the AAP refers to when it mentions the importance of early brain and child development is the attachment process of the first three to five years of life. This is the critical period when the foundation is laid in the human psyche for trust, empathy, dependency, and optimism. It is the attachment to one consistent, warm, loving, and encouraging caregiver that also ensures the development of conscience.

Anthropologists tell us that the most violent tribes are those in which infants are not touched. Neurologists tell us that holding and carrying an infant is the most important factor in the development of normal neurological functioning. Biologists tell us that the early relationship between mammals and their young is fragile.

Child Abuse and Neglect

The organization Prevent Child Abuse America, formerly the National Committee to Prevent Child Abuse, suggests that child abuse and neglect are often major contributing factors in violence among adolescents and adults.

"We'd like to think that these devastating and brutal acts of violence were unavoidable and unpredictable, but that's often not the case," said Sidney Johnson III, executive director of Prevent Child Abuse America. "Most of the time, clues suggesting possible violent behavior had been making themselves known for years."

Johnson goes on to say, "The actions of the alleged perpetrators in Colorado [and, might we say, those who bullied them] would appear to be consistent with that of children holding rage and anger from a much earlier time in their lives who haven't been able to channel it in constructive behaviors. Typically, these children lack the ability to regulate their own emotions and the ability to empathize with others, sometimes resulting in suicide, substance abuse, violent behavior and a cold indifference to other human beings."

Robin Karr-Morse, author of the 1997 book *Ghosts from the Nursery: Tracing the Roots of Violence,* said, "Media coverage of these tragedies tends to treat violent behavior as if it suddenly emerges from a developmental void. To understand the tide of violent behavior typified by this tragedy, we must look at the first 33 months of life, which harbor the seeds of violence for a growing percentage of American children."

According to Johnson, the abuse and neglect that result in violent behavior take place in families of all classes, races, and ethnicities. While many people tend to think it only happens in poor families, the emotional neglect that results in the building of such rage among our children and teens is particularly prevalent in our middle class.

Reducing Corporal Punishment

One way that we can abuse our children is by spanking them. The AAP suggests a reduction in corporal punishment as a recommended form of discipline. We cannot expect to give children the message of nonviolent problem solving if we do not practice it ourselves.

Moreover, spanking our children erodes their self-concept. Dr. Donald F. DeMoulin, a professor at the University of Tennessee and an expert in preventing violence in schools, believes that an unhealthy self-concept can lead a child down an antisocial path of destruction—from outcast to isolation to rebellion and finally, to violence.

Bullying lowers a teen's self-concept. The bully himself or

herself suffers from low self-esteem. Seeking solace from ridicule, the child associates with peers who have suffered the same fate. While this association provides the needed elevation of self-concept, it does so through negative means. The child may exhibit a brashness that may be mistaken for self-esteem, but the self-image is fed by destructive forces and is ultimately negative rather than nurturing.

According to Leon Botstein, president of Bard College, an unhealthy self-concept can be encouraged by the artificial environment of high school:

> The rules of high school turn out not to be the rules of life. Often the high school outsider becomes the more successful and admired adult. The definitions of masculinity and femininity go through sufficient transformation to make the game of popularity in high school an embarrassment. In no workplace, not even in colleges or universities, is there such a narrow segmentation by chronology.

> Given the poor quality of recruitment and training for high school teachers, it is no wonder that the curriculum and the enterprise of learning hold so little sway over young people. When puberty meets education and learning in modern America, the victory of puberty masquerading as popular culture and the tyranny of peer groups based on ludicrous values meet little resistance.

Gun Violence

How much of this violence among our teens happens in schools? According to a recent report by the Department of Education, over 6,000 students were expelled in 1996 and 1997 for bringing guns to their schools. A 1995 study by the Centers for Disease Control and Prevention (CDC) indicated that 8 percent of all students reported bringing a gun to school in a 30-day period. One handgun control organization estimates that 44 incidents of violence in US schools involving firearms were reported in the media from September 1998 through May 1999.

Is it firearms that are the problem or are teens simply more violent? There are approximately 192 million privately owned firearms in the US—65 million of which are handguns. In 1996, 10,744 people were murdered in the US; firearms were used in two out of three of those murders.

Guns kept in the home for self-protection are 43 times

more likely to kill a family member or a friend than to kill a person in self-defense. The presence of a gun in the home triples the risk of homicide in the home. The presence of a gun in the home increases the risk of suicide fivefold.

In 1995 alone, 35,957 Americans were killed with firearms (homicides, suicides, accidents). In comparison, 33,651 Americans were killed in the Korean War, while 58,148 Americans were killed in the Vietnam War.

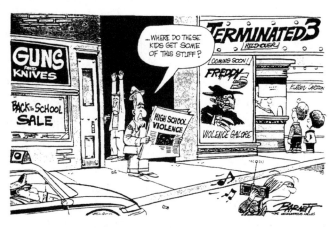

Barnett. © 1991 by *The Indianapolis News*. Reprinted with permission.

In 1994, the firearm injury death rate among males 15 to 24 years of age was 32 percent higher than the motor vehicle injury death rate. In 1995, 14 children ages 19 and under were killed with guns every day in the US.

In 1996, handguns were used to murder 2 people in New Zealand, 15 in Japan, 30 in Great Britain, 106 in Canada, 213 in Germany, and 9,390 in the US.

On April 27, 1999, then president Bill Clinton proposed gun legislation supported by the Coalition to Stop Gun Violence. The first of his proposed bills, the one requiring background checks for sales at gun shows, failed to pass the first time, but did ultimately pass because of presidential pressure. As of this writing, seven other bills remain to be passed.

Curiously, only 15 states in the US have Child Access Prevention (CAP) laws. These laws require gun owners living in households with minor children to store their guns locked and out of the reach of children. By contrast, following widespread outrage about a March 1995 shooting in Scotland in which 16 children and their teacher were killed, the British government passed a ban on handguns.

Violence in the Media

While it's obvious that the availability of guns in the US contributes to increased violence, is violence in the media also a risk factor for violence in society? According to Sylvia Ann Hewlett and Cornel West, authors of *The War Against Parents*, since 1960 more than 3,000 studies, involving almost 250,000 viewers, have evaluated television's effects on children and teenagers. The experts are in agreement. In the words of a leading researcher, Leonard Eron, "The scientific debate is over." A causal relationship between viewing violent programming and subsequent aggressive behaviors, including criminal activity, is real.

The average child watches 8,000 murders and 100,000 other acts of violence on television before entering the seventh grade. According to The Lion & Lamb Project, one long-range study involving 875 children showed that early viewing of violent television programs was positively related to later aggression—including violent criminal offenses, spousal abuse, and child abuse.

Over the years researchers have shown how a particular movie or television drama can inspire imitative or copycat behavior. In 1979, bombing and extortion threats followed the broadcast of the TV movie *Doomsday Flight*. A few years later, at least one copycat killing followed airing of *The Burning Bed*. A teenager was run over and killed, and two others were seriously injured while imitating a stunt in the 1993 movie *The Program*. John Hinkley's shooting of then president Ronald Reagan was influenced by *Taxi Driver*. And the 1994 movie *Natural Born Killers* is in a class by itself, having inspired at least 11 copycat murders.

An article in the January 1999 issue of *Pediatrics* states, "American media contribute more to adverse health outcomes than to positive or prosocial ones." A recent National Television Violence Study examined nearly 10,000 hours of television programming over a three-year period and found that 61 percent contained violence, with children's programming being the most violent.

Excessive Materialism

Evidence also suggests that many of the roots of violence in our youth, as well as the factors that put them at risk for violent behavior, are encouraged by the excesses of materialism in current US culture.

Our children are exposed to 20,000 television ads per year. There are now four 24-hour commercial channels totally devoted to children's programming. Films are peppered with advertising. In Sweden, commercials on television programming for children under 12 are prohibited by law.

Each year, teenagers view nearly 15,000 sexual references, innuendos, and jokes of which no less than 170 deal with abstinence, birth control, sexually transmitted diseases, or pregnancy. The so-called family hour of prime time television (8 to 9 p.m.) contains more than eight sexual incidents per hour, more than four times as many as in 1976.

Alcohol, tobacco, or illicit drugs are present in 70 percent of prime time network dramatic programs, 38 out of 40 top-grossing movies, and half of all music videos. Tobacco manufacturers spend $6 billion per year, and alcohol manufacturers $2 billion per year in all media, trying to entice young people to "just say yes."

As activist Ralph Nader said in a letter to Senator Trent Lott, who intends to convene a national conference on youth and culture, ". . . people in corporations are getting rich by promoting products to teenagers; corporations governed by incentives that impel them to respect no boundaries in exploiting the vulnerable minds of teenagers."

In the early 1980s, Ben Bagdikian's *The Media Monopoly* concluded that less than 50 companies had come to dominate the entirety of the US media, and as a result journalism was increasingly losing its ability to critically address the role and nature of corporate power in the US political economy. By the fourth edition of his book in 1992, mergers and acquisitions had reduced the number of dominant media firms to two dozen.

According to Robert McChesney, author of *Corporate Media and the Threat to Democracy*, since 1992 there has been an unprecedented wave of mergers and acquisitions among media giants; as a result, fewer than ten enormous vertically integrated media conglomerates now dominate US media. Time Warner, for example, the largest book and magazine publisher in the world, has annual sales of $28 billion. Time Warner owns Warner Bros., New Line Cinema, HBO, CNN, Turner Network, TNT, as well as movie theaters, retail stores, and amusement parks.

Time Warner, however, is not the largest media company in the world. This is News Corporation, whose chairman and CEO, Rupert Murdoch, is reported by *Vanity Fair* to have a net worth of $6 billion. Disney is the third media giant, with annual sales of approximately $25 billion. Viacom, owner of Nickelodeon, Simon and Schuster, Paramount, and Blockbuster, has annual sales of $6 to $13 billion. TCI, GE (NBC), Seagrams (Universal, Polygram), and Sony (Columbia, Tri-Star) complete the roster. . . .

Let's face it. We are a violent, materialistic society, and this hurts our families. What can we do to change it? First, let's not be naive any longer about the commercial interests of the gun manufacturers, the tobacco manufacturers, and the advertisers on children's programming. Let's not be naive about the special monied interests that regularly finance and influence our elected representatives.

Special interests and consumerism seduce our children and confuse their values. And they challenge the American family. Whether it's our inability to spend time with our families because of economic pressures or the commercial interests that compete for our children's attention, we have to take back control. Society may be out of control, but we must not be. We must be outraged.

Social change only happens when small, committed groups of people get together to effect change. This is the only way it ever happens. As the environmentalists say, "Think globally; act locally." Let's see what we can do.

> *"Peer pressure can have a profound impact on your physical and emotional health."*

Peer Pressure Puts Teens at Risk

Kathiann Kowalski

According to Kathiann Kowalski in the following viewpoint, peer pressure can put teenagers at risk for dangerous activities, such as drug use or shoplifting. Teenagers are particularly vulnerable to peer influences, Kowalski contends, because they are deeply affected by what others think of them. She maintains that teenagers must learn to resist negative influences and associate with peers who demonstrate positive behaviors like studying hard and volunteering. Kowalski is a contributor to *Current Health 2*, a monthly magazine that discusses teen health, social, and academic issues.

As you read, consider the following questions:

1. How does the author define peer pressure?
2. As cited by the author, what does Michael Farrell state is the best predictor of drug and alcohol abuse?
3. What are the "Four D's of Friendly Refusal," as described by Kowalski?

Kathiann Kowalski, "How Peer Pressure Can Affect You," *Current Health 2*, vol. 26, September 1999, p. 6. Copyright © 1999 by Weekly Reader Corporation. Reproduced by permission.

Erin was a sophomore from Walnut Creek, California, when she found two of her friends in the girls' room with lines of crystalline white powder all laid out. They said the white powder was "crank," a slang term for methamphetamine. "Let me try some," Erin said. That impulsive decision led Erin to a problem with addiction that eventually landed her in drug rehabilitation.

Nick came from a nice family in St. Paul, Minnesota. But that didn't keep him from hanging out with gang members. He said he enjoyed their companionship. When Nick got stabbed, however, being in the gang wasn't fun anymore.

Erin and Nick let themselves become victims of peer pressure.

Peer pressure can be deadly too. In April 1999 at Columbine High School in Littleton, Colorado, Eric Harris and Dylan Klebold, members of the Trench Coat Mafia, killed 12 fellow students, a teacher, and themselves. One possible reason for the rampage was the teasing and taunting they received as part of the Trench Coat Mafia clique—an example of peer pressure at its worst.

A Powerful Force

Peer pressure is the influence that people in your age group (your peers) exert on you. Often, the pressure includes words of encouragement, criticism, or persuasion. Or, it can be unspoken, as when group members sport similar clothes or hairstyles. Either way, peer pressure can have a profound impact on your physical and emotional health.

Why does peer pressure work so well among teens? "I think it works because kids are trying to figure out their place in their school, in their group, or whatever," observes Bernice Humphrey at Girls Incorporated's National Resource Center in Indianapolis, Indiana. "So they try to compare what they do with what other folks are doing." Teens naturally try to avoid negative attention so they won't seem weird, abnormal, or uncool. They want to fit in.

Psychologists differ on why teens are particularly prone to peer pressure. One theory says that it simply feels good to be accepted by a group, and that acceptance satisfies a need to belong. Another theory points out that life becomes easier when we act like others, or conform, rather than be different from others. Still another theory says people tend to view themselves as they think others see them, so they change to conform to others' expectations.

"Whatever the underlying motive, the effect is extremely powerful," says Robert Bornstein, a psychology professor at Miami University in Ohio. "Kids really do care what their peers think, and they really are working very hard to gain acceptance and status within the peer group."

Positive Peer Pressure

Peer pressure doesn't have to be negative. In fact, it can often be a good thing. High school senior Annie says her close friends form a loyal support system. "I know that I can always call them and tell them anything," Annie says.

Peer pressure can encourage good habits. When 14-year-old John Richards' friends play sports in Rocky River, Ohio, he feels encouraged to exercise too. "I got pressured into doing some volunteering," says 18-year-old Ariel Albores from Cleveland, Ohio. He's glad his school group involved him in community service.

Peer pressure can help give you the added strength to avoid risks to your health. Elizabeth Pozydaev, 15, from Fairview Park, Ohio, says no one in her group is into drugs. Most of her friends avoid cigarette smoking too.

Peer pressure can also encourage you to find ways to get along with others. Shouting and screaming don't resolve disputes. To get along with others, you have to know how to speak up for yourself. But you also must become skilled at resolving everyday disagreements in ways that make everyone a winner. Teens who want to keep their friends can benefit from these skills.

Risky Business

Despite the potential for good, peer pressure can have disastrous effects. "The best predictor of a kid using drugs and alcohol is what his or her friends do," says sociologist Michael Farrell at the State University of New York (SUNY) at Buffalo. The people selling drugs for the billion-dollar drug industry aren't TV stereotypes. "They're your classmates," says Farrell, "and the people using and modeling drug use are your classmates." This "in-your-face" factor produces a constant pressure that teens must deal with.

Positive Peer Pressure

When peer pressure and teenagers are mentioned in one sentence, the focus is usually on the negative affect which teenagers apparently have on each other. We are led to believe that teenagers experiment with drugs, tobacco and alcohol simply because they are afraid of not fitting in. It's like teenagers exist only in mobs and share the same opinions and do not think for themselves.

But this is not the case. Teenagers are well able to think for themselves. Indeed, one of the great advantages of peer pressure among teenagers is that it challenges teenagers to think for themselves, and not to give into the mob mentality. Peer pressure gives teenagers excellent experience in decision making. It tests their respect for authority, and for personal, family and societal values.

We are often led to believe that teenagers only encourage each other to do bad, to rebel against society. But this, again, is not true. Teenagers are always on the look out for each others' best interests. In fact, they very often generate a different kind of peer pressure, positive peer pressure. They "pressure" each other into working harder at school and at developing skills in extra-curricular activities like sport and music. This is because they realise it is important for their friends to be successful. Others take an interest in maintaining the environment and in playing a larger part in the community. In time they convince their friends to do the same.

These acts of encouragement and selflessness help to build the confidence and self-esteem of teenagers. Those who participate in the local community create a good name for themselves as trustworthy, honest, courteous, and talented individuals. Teenagers also influence each other into getting summer jobs, and thus preparing themselves for the world of work. They also earn money, much of which is for college, showing a desire to further their education.

Gerard Moloney, *Reality*, May 2000.

And when alcohol flows freely at parties, the pressure mounts to drink excessively. Binge drinking in college fraternities made national headlines in 1997 and 1998, when students died from alcohol overdoses at the Massachusetts Institute of Technology, Louisiana State University, and Case Western Reserve University.

Peer pressure can also contribute to criminal behavior. The U.S. Office of Juvenile Justice and Delinquency Prevention estimates that more than 23,000 teenage gangs roam America's cities. Some teen cliques encourage members to shoplift. Gang members are under pressure to take part in the group's violent ways. Otherwise, they risk not only alienation, but bloody retaliation.

Other risky behaviors flow from peer pressure. A study in the medical journal *Pediatrics* found that teens who became sexually active often did so because they thought it increased their status among their peers.

Academic performance also can suffer. High-achieving students hang out together at many schools, which reinforces their desire to do well. But researchers found that many students experience peer pressure to slack off at school.

Then there are potential psychological costs. "People in my neighborhood were always questioning your masculinity, your manhood—mocking you," notes Ariel. He says the rough environment where he lived was "seriously hard-core."

Even "nice" kids can get nasty. More than 70 percent of girls answering a *Teen* magazine survey said they saw clique members act mean toward outsiders. Forty percent said they personally experienced clique cruelty.

The cliques at Elizabeth's high school include a cool group, a smart group, druggies, jocks, and babes. "There are a few kids who can be really nice if you're alone with them," says Elizabeth, "but if they get with their friends, they are very careful about who they talk to and what they say. They want to be cool with their friends." To avoid being left out, clique members often tolerate or even join in group bullying. In the process, the self-esteem of the kids who give in to the pressure suffers.

When the Pressure's On

To control peer pressure, the first step is to spot it. Temptations, taunts, and threats are three ways teens can pressure each other.

1. The temptation, or "sell," tantalizes you with possible pleasures and thrills. One teen might boast how good he feels when he's high. Another teen may encourage you to come shoplifting because "we won't get caught." Someone else might suggest it would be fun to break into a home or school and destroy property.

2. Taunts include put-downs and sarcasm. "Did your mommy tell you not to drink with us?" "Are you afraid to try it?"

3. Threats of exclusion also exert pressure. "If you want to stay in our group, you'll go along," or the guilt trip: "If you were really my friend, you'd let me copy your answers."

Peer pressure also operates subtly. "The people you hang around with are going to have a profound impact on you over time," stresses Dr. Farrell. "If they're all smoking, you can say, 'Well, I'm not going to do that.' But that model and that pressure's going to be there all along."

That's what happened when Ashley's friends started smoking marijuana and drinking alcohol. She had always thought of herself as anti-drug. Over time, however, Ashley grew curious. Soon she was getting high with her friends almost every day.

Four D's of Friendly Refusal

How do you handle peer pressure? Knowing what to do about negative peer pressure can help you make good choices. Between 5,000 and 6,000 girls each year go through Girls Incorporated's Friendly PEERsuasion program. In turn, they help other kids learn how to resist negative peer pressure with the program's "Four D's of Friendly Refusal": determine, define, decide, and do.

• "The first 'D' is to determine the risk," says Bernice Humphrey. Is this trip to the mall really a shoplifting excursion? Will there be alcohol at that party? Are kids likely to use drugs when they get together after school?

• Then, define the consequences. "What are the negative things that can happen if you participate in that risky behavior?" asks Humphrey. Understanding the adverse consequences of smoking, drinking alcohol, taking drugs, engaging in risky sexual activity, and breaking the law helps you evaluate the situation. When you weigh adverse consequences against any momentary thrills, chances are you'll decide those are risks you don't want to take.

• Next, decide what you want to do right now. "Hopefully you'll replace that negative alternative with a positive option," says Humphrey. Instead of staying at a party with drinking, for example, you might catch a movie or grab a snack.

• The final "D" is having the courage to do what's best for you. Invite your friends to join you in something better, says Humphrey, but don't let their refusal deter you. If they won't join you, leave immediately.

Sharon Scott, family counselor and author of *How to Say No and Keep Your Friends*, suggests that teens have a range of possible responses beyond simply saying no and leaving the scene. Options include ignoring the offer to do something wrong, making a brief excuse, joking about it, changing the subject, or returning the challenge. If someone argues that a real friend would help him or her cheat on a test, for example, you can counter that real friends don't use pressure to make you do something wrong.

In any case, avoid long arguments. Thirty seconds is plenty of time to say no and repeat it. If other people don't get the message by then, it's their problem, not yours. Walk away.

"If you feel you don't want to do something, just stand up for yourself and say no," says Ariel. "For the most part, people respect you more if you stand up for what you believe in rather than just going along with whatever they want."

"Rely on yourself to know what's right, and don't place too much value on what your friends think," adds 18-year-old Christopher. "Hold your own ideals and values high."

Accentuate the Positive

Even before other teens try to pressure you into risky or illegal behaviors, you can take steps to control the situation. "It really does matter who you choose as your friends," says Dr. Farrell.

"The people you hang out with shape your personality," adds Annie. If you don't want to be exposed to dangerous behaviors, decide for yourself to avoid groups that do those behaviors.

"This is a good time in your life to stand up for yourself and be your own person," says Christopher. "Don't put so much emphasis on acceptance by one particular group. If they don't want to accept you, go and find your own circle of friends."

Following through on that advice is easier if you're involved in volunteer work, sports, clubs, or other activities that help you appreciate your own worth. "We need to make sure that all kids have positive experiences," says Bernice Humphrey at Girls Inc., "where they can feel confident about what they know, who they are, and their skills." These experiences help keep things in perspective when peer pressure turns negative.

Breaking away from any group can be difficult. But remember that you're not alone. A survey by The BrainWaves Group in New York City found that the majority of American teens say they enjoy learning, accept the responsibility of jobs and chores, plan to continue their education, and aim for a good career. Find other teens who model the goals and behaviors you want for yourself. As you share each other's friendship, you'll stay on track for what you really want in life.

"Gay teens dread persecution in every aspect of their lives."

Gay Teens Are at Risk

Paula Schleis and Kim Hone-McMahan

In the following viewpoint, Paula Schleis and Kim Hone-McMahan describe the risks that gay teenagers face in their schools and homes. They contend that gay teens suffer physical and verbal abuse from their peers, and, often, they risk ostracism from their families if they turn to their parents for help. Moreover, according to the authors, feelings of self-loathing and alienation often lead gay teens to attempt suicide. Schleis and Hone-McMahan are contributors to the *Akron Beacon Journal*, a newspaper in Akron, Ohio.

As you read, consider the following questions:
1. As cited by the authors, what does Karen Cimini claim causes depression in gay teenagers?
2. According to students quoted by the authors, how do teachers and administrators handle students who cast gay slurs?
3. Why do experts advise gay students to wait until they are out of high school to come out of the closet, as described by the authors?

Paula Schleis and Kim Hone-McMahan, "Gay Teens Struggle to Come to Terms with Their Sexuality, Often Battle Depression," *Akron Beacon Journal*, January 20, 1998, p. 120. Copyright © 1998 by *Akron Beacon Journal*. Reproduced by permission.

S cott's chances for having a normal, happy childhood ended the day he discovered a secret about himself.

It's a secret the 17-year-old still works diligently to bury, yet it's one that occupies his every waking moment.

You see, Scott is gay.

He didn't ask to be gay, he will tell you, and he doesn't know why he is. Who would he ask?

He's never heard a teacher explain it, and if he sought the answer in the 13-year-old health books used at Garfield High School, it would tell him he's just confused about gender roles.

His classmates? They use the term "faggot" repeatedly, tell gay jokes and taunt anyone considered "different."

His family? No way. It's clear they think homosexuality is disgusting, and a brother he loves reacts with pure hatred when the subject comes up in conversation.

His church? It's only a reminder that people think he's going to hell.

There are many people who would tell Scott being gay is as natural as being born left-handed. That many major religions no longer think it's a sin. That stories of gay couples living happy, productive lives are legion.

But Scott's closeted life has not enabled him to meet such people.

Ashamed, fearful and confused, Scott prays each night that when morning comes, he won't be gay. But he wakes after another tormented night, and nothing has changed.

There Are Others

The real shame is that Scott is not alone. Far from it.

Most surveys on the topic indicate that about 10 percent of the American population is gay. Others have challenged that statistic, saying their polls put the count at closer to 2 percent.

Many are living the same tortured existence that Scott is because as minors, they are totally dependent on the adults around them. And they see few, if any, allies among them.

Thirteen gay youths were interviewed about what it has been like growing up. Though found through a variety of sources, and representing different backgrounds and circumstances, their stories are strikingly similar.

Perhaps most alarming of all is that nine of them tried to find peace at the edge of a razor, with a handful of pills or at the end of a rope. The other four said that while they never attempted to take their lives, thoughts of suicide were never far away.

While adult gays have the freedom to seek support in adjusting to their sexual orientation, gay children are almost totally ignored—at the very time that their sexuality is developing.

"Homophobic positions kill people, literally," said Rabbi David Horowitz of Akron, Ohio, who, along with his wife, Toby, became gay activists after learning their daughter was a lesbian.

"This is not a theoretical debate. This is an issue of life and death," he said.

One expert who participated in a U.S. Department of Health and Human Services task force in 1989 concluded that nearly a third of teen suicides are committed by gay youths. Some groups have challenged that statistic as not being scientific, but no one else has attempted to conduct a similar study.

Local interviews support the idea that gay teens are living very fragile lives. Most of the teens' names in this series have been changed to protect their identity. A few even asked that their schools not be identified.

Suicide Risks

Eric, Dan, Adam, Angela, Marie and Johnnie—ages 16 through 18—all tried to take their own lives. David, 26, tried to kill himself as a teen, as did Antonio, now 23, who was hospitalized twice while in high school for attempting suicide.

Leonard Jenkins tried to hang himself when he was just 14.

Robbie Kirkland killed himself last year at age 14.

Karen Cimini, a psychologist with the Akron Family Institute, said slaying the ghosts that haunt these children is not easy.

"The depression (that they experience) is not something wrong with the brain. It's living oppressed," Cimini said. "Most of the gay people that I see are not significantly ill— they are suffering from the culture they live in."

Most of the students said their parents still don't know the source of their depression. They fear that by revealing they are gay, they risk losing the very love that is now so evident in their parents' concern for them.

While Timothy didn't act on thoughts he had of killing himself, he did do something else that is common among gay teens. He abused his body, cutting his chest, thigh and calf.

"It was a drug because, you see, physical pain stunts all of the emotional pain," explained the 17-year-old Canton Timken High School student.

Adam, a 17-year-old student in a suburban Stark County school, revealed several discolored marks on his skin and explained how he used to burn himself with matches.

Eric, 17, of Akron, used to cut himself just deep enough to draw blood. It took his mind off of what was going on in his head, he said.

Persecution at School

Gay teens dread persecution in every aspect of their lives—including family and religious institutions—but many say they feel it most acutely at school.

The teen years are a difficult time for many students. It's a time when peers become more influential than family. It's a time when children are questioning who they are and what they want to be.

And they're in a school environment that is less than kind to those deemed to be different. Something as simple as acne or a lisp will draw taunts from classmates.

Most children can take their pain home and be reassured by their parents that they are beautiful just the way they are. Historically when there's persistent abuse, parents—from African-Americans to those who have children with disabilities—have bonded together to force schools to improve the environment for their children.

Gay students, however, keep the pain to themselves. Even if their families knew what they suffered, the teens said, they feel certain their parents would be too ashamed of them to do anything about it.

So most gay teens devote their energy to hiding their sexual orientation.

They may pretend to have a steady of the opposite sex, someone who attends another school.

"When friends at school talk about what they did over the weekend, I'll say something like, 'Me and my boyfriend went to the movies,'" said Jennifer, a junior at an Akron high school.

Worse than Purgatory

Even in the best of circumstances, adolescence is a purgatory of hormonal and emotional turbulence. But for teenagers who are homosexual—and various estimates place their number at from 5 to 10 percent of U.S. high school students—it is a time of fear, shame and potentially devastating emotional hazards. According to the most comprehensive poll of randomly chosen youths—a 1995 survey of more than 4,000 students conducted by the Massachusetts Department of Education—the high school years are rife with abuse of homosexuals, some of it self-inflicted. Gay males and lesbians were five times more likely than straight kids to skip school out of fear for their safety and almost five times more likely to use cocaine. Even more alarming: According to the survey, a stunning 36.5 percent of gay and lesbian high schoolers try to kill themselves each year—this in an era when the openly gay Rupert Everett is a rising movie star and [gay music icon] Elton John practically defines middle-of-the-road pop culture.

People Weekly, August 17, 1998.

Many will date the opposite sex, but say maintaining steady relationships when there is no sexual attraction causes an anxiety of its own.

Matthew, 20, a graduate of Stow High School, said he suffered migraine headaches for a year as he tried to keep a steady girl. After they broke up, his migraines went away.

"I'm convinced not being true to myself had caused me physical pain," he said.

Missing Normal Experiences

The teens lament that they can't enjoy the normal growing-up experiences their heterosexual counterparts enjoy.

At 17, Adam has never had his first date, his first kiss.

"Seeing all of the kids at school holding hands—and having a relationship—that's really hard on me," said Adam, who described himself as a hopeless romantic. "I haven't got to experience the things you're supposed to experience as a teen."

They can't talk about their love interests, and most would never dare attend a prom or other school event with a date.

They work so hard to conceal their orientation, they can't even turn to each other for support.

There are several gay students at Garfield High School, yet when asked how many he knew, Scott said he suspected only one other.

Gay teens may appear as homophobic as any other student, laughing at gay jokes in the cafeteria or snickering when students direct the word "fag" at someone else.

And it's not always a show. Because many of the gay adults who could serve as role models are deep in their own closets, the first gay people many teens are exposed to are media stereotypes: drag queens in the movies, pedophiles in the news or flamboyant couples on talk shows.

The teens often became fearful of what they thought they had to become.

"I hated gay people," said Antonio, a graduate of Cuyahoga Falls High School. "In junior high, I even would make fun of someone who was gay to take attention away from myself."

Despite their efforts to melt into the crowd, many gay teens say classmates end up suspecting them anyway.

Eric said he suffers taunts all the time.

"They call me names and say stuff, but I just ignore them," he said.

Adam said that last year, students targeted him constantly. "They just knew that I was 'the fag,'" he said. And they reminded him five to 10 times a day, usually in the hallways between classes, and always loud enough so that everyone would hear.

Physical Abuse

Sometimes, the students said, the abuse gets physical—a shove in the hallway or a sucker punch on the way home from school—and almost always out of view of adults.

But the slurs aren't always out of adult earshot, and gay teens are acutely aware of how school staff deal with such incidents.

Teachers and administrators usually stop the use of the term "faggot" if they hear it, the students said. Officials rarely admonish a student for using the term, "That's so gay,"—meant to describe anything strange, bad or disgusting, the teens said.

Schools throughout the region reported they deal with gay slurs as they would any kind of verbal harassment. Offenders face anything from mediation to suspension, officials say.

The teachers "don't really ignore it, and they will give warnings, but that's all. They never follow through," said Scott.

What they perceive as a lack of seriousness by the adults in their schools has stopped many gay teens from confiding in counselors.

"I don't trust anyone," said Jennifer, a 16-year-old junior attending an Akron high school.

When the going gets really tough, many teens simply stay home.

Cynthia Loukas, an art teacher at Canton Timken High School, has noticed many of the young men whom she suspects are gay are repeatedly truant. "They tend to avoid the situation," she said.

And when it gets intolerable, some just drop out of school.

Johnnie, a student at Garfield High School, said classmates tormented him emotionally and physically for years. In his freshman year, he said a staff member told him that people in gym class were complaining "about a gay person changing in the same room with them."

Johnnie didn't make it through his freshman year. He dropped out of school for two years.

He has returned to Garfield and, to his surprise, has found a much-improved environment. But each day is still touch and go.

He said he'll count his blessings if he can just get through school without getting beat up. "I don't care if people don't talk to me, but don't come after me," he said.

Most of the gay teens reported being able to find a teacher they could confide in. But school officials said they were not aware of any problems facing gay students.

And in terms of curriculum, support groups or other

forms of gay awareness, a survey of districts in the five-county area revealed no district tackling the issue in any significant way.

"Has this district done anything to address an issue of this nature? No," said William Stetler, superintendent of the Lake school district in Stark County. "Has it ever come up in a meeting or discussion? No."

Akron Superintendent Brian Williams said he has never had a counselor or principal or any other staff member suggest changes in curriculum or in-service teacher training or awareness programs for students.

"I have a job that is loaded with duties . . . and you tend to put your priorities where the issues have surfaced," he said.

Garfield High School counselor Vicky Jarvie said she has had students talk with her about their sexuality, but more in terms with their home life. "They've never said they were having any big problem with the school population."

Teenage Confusion

Because most schools don't teach about what it is to be gay, their silence often fuels the confusion gay teens have about themselves.

Jennifer, 16, said she started realizing she could be attracted to females two years ago when she found herself falling in love with a girlfriend. She was confused and ashamed. She knew of a lesbian relative, so she figured it must be hereditary.

Matthew said he knew he was attracted to other boys in the fourth grade. It wasn't until high school that he realized most boys didn't feel the way he did.

"I would stay up crying at night, wondering what was wrong with me," he said. That's when high school became almost unbearable. "I couldn't wait to get out."

Change is slow, but Wooster High School Principal David Burnison said that every once in awhile, something happens to remind him there are gay teens in his school.

He recalled two girls who attended prom and took a little ribbing from a staff member who thought they were just joking. When the girls took offense, he had a talk with the staff member.

"We can't assume this is a joke," he said. The issue brought home to him the fact that "maybe we aren't as aware in the schools as we ought to be of the issues of gay students."

Burnison said he got another awareness nudge this year when he caught two girls kissing in the hallway. He said he didn't know they were both girls when he stopped them to prod them along to class, but was satisfied he handled them the way he would have handled any kids trying to sneak a kiss between classes.

Stay in the Closet

In general, experts and gay adults say they advise children to save their coming out process for adulthood and to use their teen years to learn about themselves and how to be comfortable with their sexuality.

Cimini, the psychologist, said she does more than advise.

"I tell them, beg them, plead with them, not to come out in high school, because it's dangerous," she said. "Gay bashing is primarily done by males, 16 to 19."

Even when it's not dangerous, gay teens risk losing close friends if they come out of the closet.

Antonio, the Cuyahoga Falls graduate, said he devised a little game with a close Christian friend. How would she feel if he got drunk and killed someone with a car? Could she forgive him if he had raped a girl? What would she think if he were gay?

"Being gay was worse than anything else I could dream up," he said. "It was the one thing she said she couldn't forgive. I was crushed."

Dan, 18, said when a fellow Northwest High School student forced him out last year, he tried denying it for awhile, then gave up.

"I figured I could be a gay guy and a liar, or just a gay guy," he reasoned.

His honesty cost him the friendships of all of the students in his morning prayer group. But in hindsight, that wasn't such a bad thing, he said.

Now that he's out of high school, Dan said he's been able to surround himself with people who truly care about him. He no longer takes depression medication, his suicide attempt last year is a distant memory, and he's involved in a loving relationship where both families have learned to accept him and his partner.

"I feel so much stronger now," he said.

Other teens report that when they have confided in an adult or a friend, it's had a healing effect.

Scott, the Akron Garfield student, said he felt a burden lifted when he came out to a few close friends and found acceptance.

And he noticed his personality changed. "I was always sarcastic before. I never did anything nice to anybody. I figured I was just giving them back what they gave me," he said.

Most of the students at Timothy's Stark County school know he is gay. Despite a couple of fights soon after he came out and a teacher who told him he was going to hell, he feels safe at school and finds the level of support he gets "amazing."

As a result, he said his emotional problems are "getting better by leaps and bounds."

"I'm perfectly proud of being gay," he said.

Timothy also believes that his coming out has paved the way for other gay students at his school who want the freedom to be themselves.

Glimpses of Hope

Despite the shadow they live under, many gay teens see glimpses of hope, like comedian Ellen DeGeneres coming out on her television sitcom, and the success of gay musicians like Elton John and Melissa Etheridge.

But they are equally realistic.

"Acceptance takes a long, long time," said Timothy. "I probably will never see total acceptance in my lifetime, so I'll just push for tolerance."

Antonio, 23, and Matthew, 20, represent the light at the end of their dark tunnel.

Both said their teen-age years were full of heartaches and tearful nights. Both hid their secret from close friends and family members until they were out of high school.

But as students at the University of Akron, they found support through the gay student union, they found each other, and they found the courage to come out of the closet.

Now, most members of their families accept them. Through the university group, they are helping several area teens survive their high school years.

"It seems so bad in high school, but it's gonna get better," Antonio tells those students who think they can't make it.

Periodical Bibliography

The following articles have been selected to supplement the diverse views presented in this chapter.

Sherrod Beall	"Talking with Teens: Successfully Screening for High-Risk Behavior," *Journal of the Society of Pediatric Nurses*, July–September 2000.
Erik Butler	"The New Gay Youth Revolution," *Advocate*, April 10, 2001.
Kathy Dobie	"The Only Girl in the Car: A Remembrance of Promiscuity," *Harper's*, August 1996.
Henry A. Giroux	"At War Against the Young: Corporate Culture, Schooling and the Politics of 'Zero Tolerance,'" *Against the Current*, May/June 2000.
Gayle M.B. Hanson	"Keeping the Faith, Reaching the Spirit: At-Risk Youth Programs," *Insight on the News*, March 9, 1998.
Kim Hone-McMahan and Paula Schleis	"Parents, Too, Can Have a Tough Time Dealing with a Child's Homosexuality," *Akron Beacon Journal*, January 20, 1998.
Mike Males	"The Culture War Against Kids," *Alternet*, May 22, 2001.
Don Martin and Maggie Martin	"Understanding Dysfunctional and Functional Family Behaviors for the At-Risk Adolescent," *Adolescence*, Winter 2000.
People Weekly	"Growing Up Gay," *People Weekly*, August 17, 1998.
Patrick Rogers	"Snared by the Net: Lured to the Internet by Fun and Friends, Some Teens Get Caught in a Web of Trouble," *People Weekly*, August 11, 1997.
David Whitman	"The Youth 'Crisis,'" *U.S. News & World Report*, May 5, 1997.

CHAPTER 2

How Can the Adverse Consequences of Teenage Sex and Pregnancy Be Reduced?

Chapter Preface

Unplanned teen pregnancy drastically reduces a teenager's life prospects and costs society millions of tax dollars every year. Sex educators have been searching for effective ways to reduce teen sex and pregnancy since the problem was first identified in the 1970s. For many years school-based sex education and pregnancy prevention programs concentrated more on teenage girls than on teenage boys because girls have more at stake—pregnancy—than boys do. Most programs instructed boys in the basics of sexuality and birth control, but the primary purpose of the curricula has been to influence the attitudes and behaviors of teen girls. However, recent efforts have been made to more actively include teen boys in pregnancy prevention efforts. As stated by the Urban Institute, an economic and social policy research center,

> Why males were ever excluded from the way we think about pregnancy prevention is puzzling. Sexual behavior involves two partners, and decisions to have sex and to use contraception undoubtedly reflect both partners' perspectives, whether explicitly or implicitly. Yet fertility and family are traditionally ascribed to the world of females—a perspective that has kept us from acknowledging what should have been obvious—that males must be involved in any policy solution to unintended pregnancies among teenagers.

The Urban Institute contends that teen boys are a logical target for pregnancy prevention initiatives because they initiate sex earlier than girls and tend to accumulate more sexual partners over their lifetimes.

According to the National Campaign to Prevent Teen Pregnancy (NCPTP), beginning in the 1990s, an increasing number of pregnancy prevention programs have been created that target boys and young men. Most of the programs, such as Teens on Track, Always on Saturday, Brother to Brother, and the Male Youth Enhancement Project, are community-based and target different ages and socioeconomic groups. Most of the programs try to get youths to behave responsibly, change their attitudes about women and sex, and help them develop the skills necessary to act responsibly in their relations with teenage girls. Most promote sexual abstinence, but others, assuming that most older teen boys will be sexually active, offer information about contraception. Regardless of their method, the programs strive to instill values, hopes, and ideals in teenage boys and teach them what it means to be a man and a father.

One such program, Wise Guys, was implemented in 1991 in Greensboro, North Carolina. The curriculum consists of ten components, including self-esteem, communication, sexuality, abstinence and contraception, sexually transmitted diseases, dating violence, decision-making, and parenthood. The program initially focused on pregnancy prevention, but, in response to growing incidents of date rapes on nearby campuses, recently it has given more attention to dating violence and sexual abuse. Wise Guys takes the perspective that emotional and sexual abuse can be the result of misunderstanding and poor communication. Therefore, the program encourages young men to treat girls their age as they would like their mother or sister to be treated. In addition, the program discusses goal-setting and points out to program participants that their actions now can have consequences for the future.

Evaluations of Wise Guys point to positive results. For example, one study compared 335 boys who had participated in the program to a similar group of 145 boys who had not been involved with the program. The study found that the group of boys who had participated in Wise Guys had better knowledge of sexuality and birth control, improved communication with parents, and more positive attitudes toward gender roles. Moreover, males who were sexually active when they started the program showed a 28 percent increase in contraceptive use, while the comparison group showed a decrease in contraceptive use.

The NCPTP and the Urban Institute maintain that including boys in teen pregnancy prevention efforts is crucial to reducing the incidence of unintended teen pregnancy and the spread of sexually-transmitted diseases. The authors in the following chapter debate other ways to mitigate the negative consequences of teen sex.

"Abstinence education programs for youth have been proven to be effective in reducing early sexual activity."

Abstinence-Only Sex Education Reduces Teen Sexual Activity

Robert Rector

In the following viewpoint, Heritage Foundation researcher Robert Rector argues that abstinence-based sex education programs reduce teen sexual activity and, therefore, decrease the incidence of teenage pregnancy. According to Rector, traditional "safe-sex" programs, which promote abstinence but also teach students how to avoid pregnancy and sexually transmitted diseases, implicitly condone sexual activity by instructing students in proper condom use and alternative sexual practices such as masturbation. Rector contends that abstinence-based sex education programs promote commitment, fidelity, and intimacy, which are essential to creating healthy future marriages.

As you read, consider the following questions:
1. What are three consequences of early sexual activity, according to the author?
2. What are "virginity pledge" programs, as defined by the author?
3. As cited by Rector, what were the five themes that Not Me, Not Now strove to communicate?

Robert Rector, "The Effectiveness of Abstinence Education Programs in Reducing Sexual Activity Among Youth," *Heritage Foundation Backgrounder*, April 5, 2002. Copyright © 2002 by The Heritage Foundation. Reproduced by permission.

Teenage sexual activity is a major problem confronting the nation and has led to a rising incidence of sexually transmitted diseases (STDs), emotional and psychological injuries, and out-of-wedlock childbearing. Abstinence education programs for youth have been proven to be effective in reducing early sexual activity. Abstinence programs also can provide the foundation for personal responsibility and enduring marital commitment. Therefore, they are vitally important to efforts aimed at reducing out-of-wedlock childbearing among young adult women, improving child well-being, and increasing adult happiness over the long term.

Washington policymakers should be aware of the consequences of early sexual activity, the undesirable contents of conventional "safe sex" education programs, and the findings of the professional literature concerning the effectiveness of genuine abstinence programs. In particular, policymakers should understand that:

- Sexually transmitted diseases (STDs), including incurable viral infections, have reached epidemic proportions. Annually, 3 million teenagers contract STDs; STDs afflict roughly one in four teens who are sexually active.

- Early sexual activity has multiple negative consequences for young people. Research shows that young people who become sexually active are not only vulnerable to STDs, but also likely to experience emotional and psychological injuries, subsequent marital difficulties, and involvement in other high-risk behaviors.

- Conventional "safe sex" programs (sometimes erroneously called "abstinence plus" programs) place little or no emphasis on encouraging young people to abstain from early sexual activity. Instead, such programs strongly promote condom use and implicitly condone sexual activity among teens. Nearly all such programs contain material and messages that would be alarming and offensive to the overwhelming majority of parents.

- Despite claims to the contrary, there are 10 scientific evaluations showing that real abstinence programs can be highly effective in reducing early sexual activity. Moreover, real abstinence education is a fairly young field; thus, the number of evaluations of abstinence programs at present is somewhat limited. In the near future, many additional evaluations that demonstrate the effectiveness of abstinence education will become available.

Consequences of Early Sexual Activity

Young people who become sexually active enter an arena of high-risk behavior that leads to physical and emotional damage. Each year, influenced by a combination of a youthful assumption of invincibility and a lack of guidance (or misguidance and misleading information), millions of teens ignore those risks and suffer the consequences.

Sexually Transmitted Diseases

The nation is experiencing an epidemic of sexually transmitted diseases that is steadily expanding. In the 1960s, the beginning of the "sexual revolution," the dominant diseases related to sexual activity were syphilis and gonorrhea. Today, there are more than 20 widespread STDs, infecting an average of more than 15 million individuals each year. Two-thirds of all STDs occur in people who are 25 years of age or younger. Each year, 3 million teens contract an STD; overall, one-fourth of sexually active teens have been afflicted.

There is no cure for sexually transmitted viral diseases such as the human immunodeficiency virus (HIV) and herpes, which take their toll on people throughout life. Other common viral STDs are the Human Papillomavirus (HPV)—the leading viral STD, with 5.5 million cases reported each year, and the cause of nearly all cases of cervical cancer that kill approximately 4,800 women per year—and *Chlamydia trachomatis*, which is associated with pelvic inflammatory disease that scars the fallopian tubes and is the fastest growing cause of infertility.

Significantly, research shows that condom use offers relatively little protection (from "zero" to "some") for herpes and no protection from the deadly HPV. A review of the scientific literature reveals that, on average, condoms failed to prevent the transmission of the HIV virus—which causes the immune deficiency syndrome known as AIDS—between 15 percent and 31 percent of the time. It should not be surprising, therefore, that while condom use has increased over the past 25 years, the spread of STDs has likewise continued to rise.

Emotional and Psychological Injury

Young people who become sexually active are vulnerable to emotional and psychological injury as well as to physical diseases. Many young girls report experiencing regret or guilt after their initial sexual experience. In the words of one psychiatrist who recalls the effects of her own sexual experimentation in her teens, "The longest-standing, deepest wound I gave myself was heartfelt; that sick, used feeling of having given a precious part of myself—my soul—to so many and for nothing, still aches. I never imagined I'd pay so dearly and for so long."

Sexually active youth often live with anxiety about the possibility of an unwanted pregnancy or contracting a devastating STD. Those who do become infected with a disease suffer emotional as well as physical effects. Fears regarding the course of the disease are coupled with a loss of self-esteem and self-confidence. In a survey by the Medical Institute for Sexual Health, 80 percent of those who had herpes said that they felt "less confident" and "less desirable sexually."

In addition, early sexual activity can negatively affect the ability of young people to form stable and healthy relationships in a later marriage. Sexual relationships among teenagers are fleeting and unstable, and broken intimate relationships can have serious long-term developmental effects. A series of broken intimate relationships can undermine an individual's capacity to enter into a committed, loving marital relationship. In general, individuals who engage in premarital sexual activity are 50 percent more likely to divorce later in life than those who do not. Divorce, in turn, leads to sharp reductions in adult happiness and child well-being.

Marital relationships that follow early sexual activity can also suffer from the emotional impact of infertility resulting from an STD infection, ranging from a sense of guilt to depression. In the words of one gynecologist and fertility specialist, "Infertility is so devastating, it often disorients my patients to life itself. This is more than shock or even depression. It impacts every level of their lives, including their marriage.". . .

Out-of-Wedlock Childbearing

Today, it is widely reported that one child in three is born out of wedlock. Only 14 percent of these births occur to women under the age of 18. Most occur to women in their early twenties. Thus, giving birth control to teens in high school through safe-sex programs will have little effect on out-of-wedlock childbearing.

Nearly half of the mothers who give birth outside marriage are cohabiting with the child's father at the time of birth. These fathers, like the mothers, are typically in their early twenties. Out-of-wedlock childbearing is, thus, not the result of teenagers' lack of knowledge about birth control or a lack of availability of birth control. Rather, it is part of a crisis in the relationships of young adult men and women. Out-of-wedlock childbearing, in most cases, occurs because young adult men and women are unable to develop committed, loving marital relationships. Abstinence programs, therefore, which focus on developing loving and enduring relationships and preparation for successful marriages, are an essential first step in reducing future levels of out-of-wedlock births.

The Silent Scandal: Promoting Teen Sex

With millions of dollars in sex-education programs at stake, it is not surprising that the groups that have previously dominated the arena have taken action to block the growing movement to abstinence-only education. Such organizations, including the Sexuality Information and Education Council of the United States (SIECUS), Planned Parenthood, and the National Abortion and Reproductive Rights Action League (NARAL), have been prime supporters of "safe-sex" programs for youth, which entail guidance on the use of condoms and other means of contraception while giving a condescending nod to abstinence. Clearly, the caveat that says "and if you do engage in sex, this is how you should do it" substantially weakens an admonition against early non-marital sexual activity.

Not only do such programs, by their very nature, minimize the abstinence component of sex education, but many of these programs also effectively promote sexual activity among the youths they teach. Guidelines developed by SIECUS, for example, include teaching children aged 5 through 8 about masturbation and teaching youths aged 9 through 12 about alternative sexual activities such as mutual masturbation, "outercourse," and oral sex. In addition, the SIECUS guidelines suggest informing youths aged 16 through 18 that sexual activity can include bathing or showering together as well as oral, vaginal, or anal intercourse, and that they can use erotic photographs, movies, or literature to enhance their sexual fantasies when alone or with a partner. Not only do such activities carry their own risks for youth, but they are also likely to increase the incidence of sexual intercourse.

Abstinence Programs Work

It is . . . likely that the growth of privately funded abstinence programs have been, at least in part, responsible for the improvement in the [decline in teenage pregnancy].

- The growth of the abstinence-only message coincides with the improvement in the data reflecting adolescent sexual behavior.
- Scientific research demonstrates that abstinence programs are effective.
- Between 1982 and 1987 a community abstinence message implemented in Denmark, South Carolina reduced teen pregnancy by 59 percent.
- Inner city students in the Best Friends program in Washington, DC, were reported to have a pregnancy rate of only 1.1 percent compared to an overall city pregnancy rate among high school aged females of 26 percent.
- A study in the *Journal of the American Medical Association* entitled "Add Health" reported that the factor most associated with a delay in early sexual onset was a pledge of virginity. The virginity pledge is a foundational aspect of the True Love Waits abstinence program.

Abbylin Sellers, *Focus on the Family*, May 1998.

In recent years, parental support for real abstinence education has grown. Because of this, many traditional safe-sex programs now take to calling themselves "abstinence plus" or "abstinence-based" education. In reality, there is little abstinence training in "abstinence-based" education. Instead, these programs are thinly disguised efforts to promote condom use. The actual content of most "abstinence plus" curricula would be alarming to most parents. For example, such programs typically have condom use exercises in which middle school students practice unrolling condoms on cucumbers or dildoes.

Effective Abstinence Programs

Critics of abstinence education often assert that while abstinence education that exclusively promotes abstaining from premarital sex is a good idea in theory, there is no evidence that such education can actually reduce sexual activity among young people. Such criticism is erroneous. There are currently 10 scientific evaluations ([five of which are] described below) that demonstrate the effectiveness of abstinence programs in altering sexual behavior. Each of the programs evaluated is a real abstinence (or what is conventionally termed an "abstinence only") program; that is, the program does not provide contraceptives or encourage their use.

[Five of] the abstinence programs and their evaluations are as follows:

1. *Virginity Pledge Programs.* An article in the *Journal of the American Medical Association* by Dr. Michael Resnick and others entitled "Protecting Adolescents From Harm: Findings from the National Longitudinal Study on Adolescent Health" shows that "abstinence pledge" programs are dramatically effective in reducing sexual activity among teenagers in grades 7 through 12. Based on a large national sample of adolescents, the study concludes that "Adolescents who reported having taken a pledge to remain a virgin were at significantly lower risk of early age of sexual debut."

   In fact, the study found that participating in an abstinence program and taking a formal pledge of virginity were by far the most significant factors in a youth delaying early sexual activity. The study compared students who had taken a formal pledge of virginity with students who had not taken a pledge but were otherwise identical in terms of race, income, school performance, degree of religiousness, and other social and demographic factors. Based on this analysis, the authors discovered that the level of sexual activity among students who had taken a formal pledge of virginity was one-fourth the level of that of their counterparts who had not taken a pledge. Overall, nearly 16 percent of girls and 10 percent of boys were found to have taken a virginity pledge.

2. *Not Me, Not Now*. Not Me, Not Now is a community-wide abstinence intervention targeted to 9- to 14-year-olds in Monroe County, New York, which includes the city of Rochester. The Not Me, Not Now program devised a mass communications strategy to promote the abstinence message through paid TV and radio advertising, billboards, posters distributed in schools, educational materials for parents, an interactive Web site, and educational sessions in school and community settings. The program sought to communicate five themes: raising awareness of the problem of teen pregnancy, increasing an understanding of the negative consequences of teen pregnancy, developing resistance to peer pressure, promoting parent-child communication, and promoting abstinence among teens.

Not Me, Not Now was effective in reaching early teen listeners, with some 95 percent of the target audience within the county reporting that they had seen a Not Me, Not Now ad. During the intervention period, the program achieved a statistically significant positive shift in attitudes among pre-teens and early teens in the county. The sexual activity rate of 15-year-olds across the county (as reported in the Youth Risk Behavior Survey) dropped by a statistically significant amount from 46.6 percent to 31.6 percent during the intervention period. Finally, the pregnancy rate for girls aged 15 through 17 in Monroe County fell by a statistically significant amount, from 63.4 pregnancies per 1,000 girls to 49.5 pregnancies per 1,000. The teen pregnancy rate fell more rapidly in Monroe County than in comparison counties and in upstate New York in general, and the difference in the rate of decrease was statistically significant.

3. *Operation Keepsake*. Operation Keepsake is an abstinence program for 12- and 13-year-old children in Cleveland,

Ohio. Some 77 percent of the children in the program were black or Hispanic. An evaluation of the program in 2001, involving a sample of over 800 students, found that "Operation Keepsake had a clear and sustainable impact on . . . abstinence beliefs." The evaluation showed that the program reduced the rate of onset of sexual activity (loss of virginity) by roughly two-thirds relative to comparable students in control schools who did not participate in the program. In addition, the program reduced by about one-fifth the rate of current sexual activity among those with prior sexual experience.

4. *Abstinence by Choice.* Abstinence by Choice operates in 20 schools in the Little Rock area of Arkansas. The program targets 7th, 8th, and 9th grade students and reaches about 4,000 youths each year. A recent evaluation, involving a sample of nearly 1,000 students, shows that the program has been highly effective in changing the attitudes that are directly linked to early sexual activity. Moreover, the program reduced the sexual activity rates of girls by approximately 40 percent (from 10.2 percent to 5.9 percent) and the rate for boys by approximately 30 percent (from 22.8 percent to 15.8 percent) when compared with similar students who had not been exposed to the program. (The sexual activity rate of students in the program was compared with the rate of sexual activity among control students in the same grade in the same schools prior to the commencement of the program.)

5. *Virginity Pledge Movement.* A 2001 evaluation of the effectiveness of virginity pledge movement using data from the National Longitudinal Study of Adolescent Health finds that virginity pledge programs are highly effective in helping adolescents to delay sexual activity. According to the authors of the study:

> Adolescents who pledge, controlling for all of the usual characteristics of adolescents and their social contexts that are associated with the transition to sex, are much *less* likely than adolescents who do not pledge, to have intercourse. The delay effect is substantial and robust. Pledging delays intercourse for a long time.

The study, based on a sample of more than 5,000 students, concludes that taking a virginity pledge reduces by one-third the probability that an adolescent will begin sexual activity compared with other adolescents of the same gender and age, after controlling for a host of other factors linked to sexual activity rates such as physical maturity, parental disapproval of sexual activity, school achievement, and race. When taking a virginity pledge is combined with strong parental disapproval of sexual activity, the probability of initiation of sexual activity is reduced by 75 percent or more. . . .

Commitment, Fidelity, and Intimacy

Real abstinence education is essential to reducing out-of-wedlock childbearing, preventing sexually transmitted diseases, and improving emotional and physical well-being among the nation's youth. True abstinence education programs help young people to develop an understanding of commitment, fidelity, and intimacy that will serve them well as the foundations of healthy marital life in the future.

Abstinence education programs have repeatedly been shown to be effective in reducing sexual activity among their participants. However, funding for the evaluation of abstinence education programs until very recently has ranged from meager to non-existent. Currently, the number of adequately funded evaluations of abstinence education is increasing. At present, there are several promising new evaluations nearing completion. As each year passes, it can be expected that the number of evaluations showing that abstinence education does significantly reduce sexual activity will grow steadily.

Abstinence education is a nascent and developing field. Substantial funding for abstinence education became available only within the past few years. As abstinence programs develop and become more broadly available, future evaluations will enable the programs to hone and increase their effectiveness.

"There is no scientific evidence that abstinence-only curricula in schools are effective, either in delaying onset of first intercourse or preventing pregnancies and STDs."

Abstinence-Only Sex Education Is Ineffective

Deborah M. Roffman

In the following viewpoint, Deborah M. Roffman argues that abstinence-only sex education programs are unrealistic because they fail to properly educate teens in how to protect themselves form the risks of sexual activity. Moreover, she maintains that abstinence-only programs try to control teenagers by telling them what to do, an approach that alienates many teens and encourages them to engage in the very activities such programs are designed to discourage. In contrast, comprehensive sex education programs respect teens' growing autonomy by encouraging them to think and make informed decisions about sex, Roffman claims. Roffman is a sex educator and the author of *Sex and Sensibility: The Thinking Parent's Guide to Talking Sense About Sex*.

As you read, consider the following questions:
1. Why did the author refuse to participate in a radio debate about sex education?
2. How do the arguments in the sex education debate only "serve the needs of adults," according to Roffman?

As a sexuality educator, I felt my spirits lift in June 2001 when Surgeon General David Satcher issued his "Call to Action" on sexual health. In this groundbreaking report, the nation's chief doctor made the case for a comprehensive approach to sex education in the schools, combining an emphasis on abstinence with information on preventing pregnancy and sexually transmitted diseases. Here at last, I allowed myself to hope, was an event that could stimulate an unprecedented national dialogue on an issue that hits us where it matters most—the lives and health of our children.

Then, within a day, the George W. Bush administration distanced itself from the report, and conservatives began to talk about a replacement for Satcher. The White House made clear that it would aggressively seek to increase funding for public school "abstinence-only" programs, which by statute prohibit discussion of other methods of disease and pregnancy prevention.

And I thought, here we go again.

Abstinence Wars

Welcome to the latest skirmish in the nation's "abstinence wars." This fierce subsidiary of the much touted "culture wars" has stalled realistic and creative policy-making in the field of sex education for more than three decades. Satcher's attempt notwithstanding, it became clear to me that we weren't about to make any progress soon when I received a call asking me to participate in a Baltimore talk-radio program. The topic: "Traditional approaches to sex education vs. the abstinence-until-marriage approach."

No, thanks, I said, as I always do whenever the issue is framed in this way. That's because I believe that pitching comprehensive sex education as the opposite, in fact the enemy, of abstinence is false, misleading and counterproductive, and that as long as we in the United States continue to polarize this issue, we're kidding ourselves if we think we're doing well by our kids.

Despite the fact that more than 80 percent of American adults say they favor a comprehensive approach to sex education, this either/or standoff persists. What is the justification for it? Abstinence-only proponents argue that giving a clear and unequivocal directive is the best and most effective strategy. Adults must insist that refraining from sex until marriage is the only safe and moral course; providing additional information about protection lends unacceptable credibility to any other choice. In any case, they say, the need for such information becomes moot, because kids who abstain will not be putting themselves in a situation where they need protection.

Clear and Informed Messages

But there's something missing from this argument. Adolescents need clear messages—most definitely—but as my experience over more than 30 years in the classroom has taught me, clarity by itself is never enough. Consider this example. Some time ago, a nationally prominent abstinence-only educator came to the all-girls school where I teach, one that works particularly hard at turning out girls who are skilled critical thinkers. The woman gave the girls unequivocal messages about how damaging premarital intercourse would be in their lives, but her moralizing tone infuriated many of the eighth-graders who heard her presentation. By the time they came to my class, they were ready to kill the messenger—and her messages. Said one student: "There will be girls who go out and 'do it' just to spite her!"

Once I got the girls to settle down and refocus, I was able to reframe the conversation in a manner that felt more respectful. "If you were presenting the abstinence argument, what would you say, and how would you say it?" I asked. From then on, these 13- and 14-year-olds were more than able on their own to articulate and seriously consider all of the points the speaker had been trying to make. "Contraceptives might not work 100 percent," one said, "and a baby would change your whole life." Added another, "Even if you were able to avoid physical effects, we're too young to handle the emotions."

The students even made some excellent points the speaker had not brought up, based on their own life experiences. One, for instance, noted that boys usually aren't as socially mature as girls, and might not want the same things from a relationship. The girl next to her nodded and added,

"Besides, if you had to hide things you were doing from your parents, you wouldn't feel good about yourself." I remember driving home that day and thinking to myself: How ironic.

Causing Trouble

Here are a few examples of the problems created by the abstinence-only approach to sexuality "education":

- *Public funds go to religious institutions for* anti-*sexuality education*. In Montana, the Catholic diocese of Helena received $14,000 from the state's Department of Health & Human Services for classes in the "Assets for Abstinence." In Louisiana, a network of pastors is bringing the abstinence-only message to religious congregations with public funds, and the Governor's Program on Abstinence is appointing regional coordinators and other staff members from such religious organizations as the Baptist Collegiate Ministries, Rapides Station Community Ministries, Diocese of Lafayette, Revolution Ministries, Caring to Love Ministries, All Saints Crusade Foundation, Concerned Christian Women of Livingston, Catholic Charities, Christian Counseling Center, and Community Christian Concern.

- *Public schools host "chastity" events.* In California, Pennsylvania, Alabama, and many other states, schools regularly host chastity pledges and rallies on school premises during school hours. During these rituals, students often pledge "to God" that they will remain abstinent until they marry.

- *Textbooks are censored.* The school board in Franklin County, North Carolina, ordered three chapters literally sliced out of a ninth-grade health textbook because the material did not adhere to state law mandating abstinence-only education. The chapters covered AIDS and other sexually transmitted infections, marriage and partnering, and contraception. In Lynchburg, Virginia, school board members refused to approve a high school science textbook unless an illustration of a vagina was covered or cut out.

- *Crucial health programs are canceled.* In response to a petition from 28 parents, a highly regarded, comprehensive, AIDS-prevention presentation for high school students in the Syracuse, New York, area, given by the local AIDS Task Force, was canceled for future students. In Illinois, critics blasted a U.S. Centers for Disease Control and Prevention program, called "Reducing the Risk," because they claim it is inconsistent with an abstinence-only message.

National Coalition Against Censorship, "Abstinence-Only Education: Why First Amendment Supporters Should Oppose It," September 2001.

I—the supposed "anti-abstinence" lady, because I also talk about contraception and STD prevention—had saved the day for the abstinence message!

In truth, the kinds of false polarities that have been set up in the sex education debate only serve the needs of adults. They enable politicians who hold up the pro-abstinence/anti-education banner, for example, to sound noble and moral and to give the appearance that their side is holding down the fort at the entrance to the moral high ground. And this tactic is neither liberal nor conservative, Democratic nor Republican: Federal involvement in promoting abstinence-only education—$250 million in matching funds to the states—was originally signed into law in 1996 on the watch of the Bill Clinton administration.

Harsh Realities

Regardless of our personal politics, the guidance we deliver our young people must take into account the harsh realities of adolescent sexual health in this country today: Every year, nearly 10 percent of teenage girls become pregnant; teens acquire an estimated 3 million sexually transmitted infections every year; 25 percent of new HIV cases occur in people under the age of 20; 50 percent of all 9th- through 12th-grade students have already had sexual intercourse.

There is no scientific evidence that abstinence-only curricula in schools are effective, either in delaying onset of first intercourse or preventing pregnancy and STDs. On the other hand, multiple studies show that the combination of a strong abstinence message and information about methods of protection does work and therefore makes the most logical sense.

My guess as to why it works is that the underlying message is the developmentally correct one. The message communicated to teenagers is that we adults recognize them as maturing individuals who are learning to take responsibility for themselves, and that we will not treat them as though they lack the ability to reason on their own. We can tell them that we will do our very best to provide appropriate limits and help guide their choices, but we know that we cannot ultimately make all of those choices for them.

This is an approach that adolescents will hear—and buy. We can all remember from our own adolescence how teenagers resist and resent adults who attempt to control their lives, but respect those who set clear limits while showing respect for them and their developing sense of autonomy.

Teaching Teens to Think

It's ironic, and frightening to me as an educator, that the underlying message in the abstinence-only approach is actually the same as the one young people get from the popular media. The words sound diametrically opposed ("Don't do it!" vs. "Do it now!") but the underlying message is exactly the same: "When it comes to sex, there's nothing for you to think about." In neither case are we training teenagers to do what they must learn to do for themselves: Think. Here's what I aim for in my classrooms: teenagers with lightbulbs over their heads and a look in their eyes that says, "This issue is a lot more complicated than I realized. I'd better think this one through very carefully."

Thinking responsibly and correctly about an issue as complicated as sex is hard. Quite frankly, adults have difficulty thinking through all that it entails themselves, let alone helping kids do so. Too many of us are tempted to hide behind the false argument that talking about abstinence and condoms amounts to sending a mixed message. "Wait!" and "Protect yourself!" are not mixed messages. Both are about protection. If it sounds like a mixed message when it comes out of our mouths, we need to keep fixing it until it's clear.

What I know from listening to thousands of parents over the years is that all of them love their children and want them to become prudent, caring, ethical and fulfilled people. All want their children eventually to embrace their sexuality and learn to enjoy it as a positive life force. And all want their children to understand that sexual behavior, especially sexual intercourse, is extraordinarily powerful, and that only people who are capable of mature, responsible conduct should ever consider engaging in it.

These are immensely important shared values, the enormous and fertile common ground upon which we all stand, even as our areas of disagreement may blind us to it.

Perceptions of Abstinence

Many parents view abstinence as an issue of postponement; they want their children to abstain at least until they are developmentally ready and want schools to help make them ready for that time. Others view abstinence as an end in itself, and sex as something to be reserved for the holy sacrament of marriage; they want assurance that schools will present that, too, as a legitimate and viable option.

But promoting abstinence as the only option is to negate the critical needs of millions of young people, the wishes of the majority of American parents, and the universality of our fundamental hopes and dreams for our children.

"The teen pregnancy 'crisis' is less a crisis of pregnancy than an epidemic of young, unwed motherhood."

Teenage Parents Should Get Married

Dana Mack

According to Dana Mack in the following viewpoint, encouraging teenage parents to marry could alleviate the problems associated with teenage childbearing, such as poverty and welfare dependency. Mack argues that early motherhood, not marriage, often harms the educational and career prospects of young women. She contends that marriage offers more financial and emotional stability to the mother and her child than does single-parenthood. Mack is the author of *The Assault on Parenthood: How Our Culture Undermines the Family.*

As you read, consider the following questions:

1. What is the main difference between teenage pregnancy today and in the early 1970s, according to Mack?
2. As stated by the author, how do adults give ambivalent messages about the importance of marriage?
3. According to Mack, why is marriage often the only chance a mother will have to provide her child with a loving and supportive father?

Dana Mack, "Commentary; Teenage Mothers Should Get Married; Values: Discouraging Such Marriages Virtually Assures Children of a Life of Poverty," *Los Angeles Times*, October 1999, p. 7. Copyright © 1999 by Los Angeles Times Syndicate. Reproduced by permission.

Despite nearly 40 years of consistent efforts by government, schools, social services and the medical community, the United States still faces insupportable levels of teen childbearing. Our teen birth rate is nine times higher than the Netherlands', four times higher than Sweden's and 65% higher than Britain's. What is to be done about it? A 1999 report issued by the Institute for American Values, a New York–based family and social policy research organization, suggests that the worst social effects of teen childbearing could largely disappear—if only we rethink our approach to the problem.

Mothers Without Marriage

Maggie Gallagher, an affiliate scholar of the institute, has produced a comprehensive review and critique of the social science research on teen pregnancy, titled "The Age of Unwed Mothers."

In an unusual and provocative take on the subject, Gallagher suggests that the real problem with teen childbearing today is that teenage mothers are not marrying the fathers of their children.

Gallagher's assertion gives us pause for thought.

Levels of teen childbearing are actually no higher today than they were in the early 1970s. The principal difference between the early 1970s and today is that more and more childbearing teens decline to legitimize their pregnancies and births. Since that time, the percentage of teenage girls conceiving out of wedlock who married the fathers of their children fell from 47% to 16%.

Indeed, what many refer to as the teen pregnancy "crisis" is less a crisis of pregnancy than an epidemic of young, unwed motherhood.

This epidemic, unfortunately, has been aggravated by educators and pregnancy counselors who discourage even 18- and 19-year-olds who decide to carry their pregnancies to term from marrying.

Ambivalent Messages

Apparently, we adults are sending ambivalent messages about the importance of marriage to the well-being of children.

Not only are we often unwilling to express social disapproval of teen sex and unwed motherhood; in the errant belief that teenage marriages are bound to fail, we are all too silent on the advantages marriage may bring to teen mothers.

Teen marriages are more vulnerable to divorce than marriages of women in their mid-20s. But about half of the marriages of 18- and 19-year-olds succeed. And teen marriages involving children actually have a better chance at success than marriages that do not involve children.

Tellingly, when teen mothers do not marry the fathers of their children, they are more likely in their 20s to be poor and welfare-dependent, and they are less likely, ultimately, to marry at all.

Percent of Premaritally Pregnant Women Aged 15–19 Marrying Before the Birth of Their First Child, 1930–1994

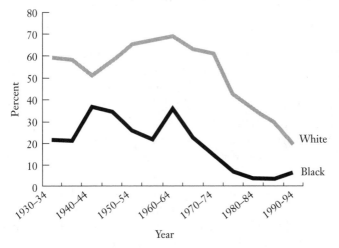

Amara Bachu, 1999, based on U.S. Census Bureau data.

Research indicates that it is primarily early motherhood, not marriage, that derails the educational and work attainment of young women. However dark the prospects of the most hasty teen marriage, that marriage is often the only chance a teenage mother will get to give her child the love and material benefits of a committed father.

Gallagher contends that the somewhat superficial prejudice of educators, social service professionals and counselors against early marriage has profoundly affected the teenage mind-set.

In interviews with young unwed mothers, she often heard the refrain: "I'd like to marry eventually, but I'm still too young." Old enough to assume the heavy responsibilities of motherhood, but too young to marry?

It appears we must address profound deficiencies in the way we talk to young people about marriage and the family. Increasingly, our youth seem to be picking up the message that while marriage may demand maturity, parenting does not; and that marriage and children are totally separate and unrelated spheres of life.

Can childbearing and child-rearing really have nothing to do with any relationship between a man and a woman that might lead them to formally unite their lives?

Questionable Fathers

Granted, many teenage girls who bear children have been impregnated by men whose prospects as both husbands and fathers are less than desirable. Yet we must do what we can, when appropriate, to get older teenagers who are determined to keep their babies to consider the option of marriage. And we must take steps to support teenage marriages with at least some of the community resources we now devote exclusively to single teen mothers.

The "M" word, marriage, is not a word without dignity and worth. It is a word that for children of teenagers might mean the difference between lives of emotional and economic scarcity and lives of relative security.

"Marriages among teenagers are notoriously unstable."

Encouraging Marriage Does Not Solve the Problems Associated with Teenage Pregnancy

Isabel V. Sawhill

In the following viewpoint, Isabel V. Sawhill argues that encouraging teenage parents to marry will not solve the problems associated with teen pregnancy. She grants that children fare better when their parents are married than when they are not married, but notes that teenage marriages have an extremely high failure rate. In addition, she claims that by focusing their efforts on getting teen parents to wed, government programs fail to address why teenagers get pregnant in the first place. The best way to reduce the problems associated with teenage pregnancy, according to Sawhill, is to encourage abstinence, but also to teach teens about birth control. Sawhill is a senior fellow at the Brookings Institute, a liberal research and educational organization.

As you read, consider the following questions:
1. What does Sawhill mean when she claims that the issue of unwed pregnancy is timing?
2. As cited by the author, what did Daniel Lichter's research conclude about young men?
3. What two reasons does Sawhill give to be optimistic about teenage pregnancy?

Isabel V. Sawhill, "Is Lack of Marriage the Real Problem?" *American Prospect*, vol. 13, April 8, 2002. Copyright © 2002 by *American Prospect*. Reproduced by permission.

Marriage is now a hot topic in Washington policy circles. Ensuring that more children are born and raised within marriage is, in my view, a worthy objective. Marriage as a value has begun to disappear from the cultural lexicon, and affirmative efforts to underscore its importance, especially to children, should not be dismissed. But this begs the question of what states or the federal government realistically can do to promote it.

The problem is not that people don't marry. Ninety percent of all American women are married by the age of 45. The problem is early childbearing. Until they are in their mid-twenties, more women have had babies than have married. After the mid-twenties, the numbers reverse. The issue, then, is timing. We don't need to encourage more people to marry unless our goal is to reach 100 percent married (which, incidentally, would require that we legalize same-sex marriages). What we need instead is to stop people from having babies before they get married. Most of these births are unintended and most are the result of early unprotected sex.

Start with Teenagers

The place to start, obviously, is with teenagers. Although only 30 percent of all out-of-wedlock births are to teens, half of *first* out-of-wedlock births are to women under the age of 20. Having had a first baby outside marriage, these teens often drop out of school, go on welfare, and have additional children in their twenties without marrying. In other words, the problem isn't limited to teens but it typically begins in the teenage years. And these families started by a teen mother are the ones most at risk of long-term poverty and a host of other problems.

Will more marriage solve this problem? Hardly. Marriages among teenagers are notoriously unstable. In addition, once a woman has become a single mother, her chances of marrying anyone other than the father of her child are greatly reduced. New research by sociology professor Daniel Lichter shows that this failure to marry is mostly a result of the presence of children rather than the characteristics of the mothers themselves. It seems obvious, but marriage advocates seem not to have noticed that young men are reluctant to take responsibility for someone else's child. William Julius Wilson long ago popularized the notion that the absence of marriageable males in many distressed urban black communities inhibits marriage. What Lichter is finding is that there's a shortage of marriageable females in general.

Better-educated women are increasingly delaying both marriage and childbearing until they are in their mid- to late-twenties and even older. This pattern is consistent with spending more time in school and with establishing a career path before taking on family responsibilities. Our goal should be to help less-educated women follow a similar path. The alternative—to encourage girls in their teens or early twenties to marry—is not consistent with society's interest in encouraging people to acquire the skills needed in the new economy or with the job opportunities available to today's young women.

Moreover, older parents are usually better parents, so this strategy would work to improve child well-being. And later marriages are much more stable. So if we want to discourage divorce, this makes sense as well. Indeed, age at marriage is the primary predictor of marital stability.

Reasons for Optimism

If early childbearing is the problem, what is the solution? Haven't efforts to reduce teen pregnancies and births been a failure? Ten years ago the answer to this question might have been yes. But there are now reasons for much greater optimism. First of all, teen pregnancies and birthrates have declined sharply in the 1990s. Between 1991 and 2000, the teen birthrate declined 22 percent to 48.5 births per 1,000 females 15 to 19 years old. (The declines were especially sharp for black teens.) Because so many of these teen births are to unmarried women, this decline has contributed very directly to a leveling off of the proportion of all children born outside marriage in the late 1990s.

But there is a second reason to be optimistic. Recent research has found a number of programs that effectively prevent teen pregnancies. These include sex-education programs that encourage abstinence but also teach about birth control, and youth-development programs such as after-school mentoring or community service. Another promising approach is public-service ad campaigns that use the power of the media to reach large numbers of teens in a way that will never be possible through community-based efforts or classroom instruction alone.

Teen Marriages Are Risky

It is likely that, as with all women, teens experience some current economic benefit from being married. However, there are a number of important reasons to question an assumption that a teen mother who is not inclined to marry would be better off married. Notably, high rates of dissolution of teen marriages may make marriage a riskier bet for teen women's long-term economic security than it is for older women. Since married teens are more likely to have a rapid repeat birth and this can affect school completion, marriage may hamper future economic stability. The high rates of abuse by intimates that young women experience suggest yet another reason to be cautious.

For those teens who do marry, we urge policymakers to provide support services to help them build strong relationships. However, the instability of teen marriage and the risks it can pose should give pause to any policymaker who is eager to encourage pregnant adolescents to walk down the aisle.

Naomi Seiler, "Is Teen Marriage a Solution?" Center for Law and Social Policy, April 2002.

Conservatives want to reduce early out-of-wedlock pregnancies by funding "abstinence only" education programs. The George W. Bush administration's budget proposes to increase funding for these from $102 million to $135 million. These programs have not been adequately evaluated and, so far, their effectiveness has not been proven. That doesn't mean that encouraging abstinence is a bad idea. Teen-pregnancy rates dropped in the 1990s because of more abstinence and more or better use of birth control. Nor does it mean that encouraging people to delay childbearing until they are married is a bad idea. But government programs and sex-education curricula dictated from Washington are not the best way of achieving these goals. Instead, we should focus on empowering parents, schools, and nonprofit organizations, including those that are religiously affiliated, to send the message that children are better off with two committed parents who are married to each other. That means delaying unprotected sex and unwanted births.

Government Efforts

Given these facts, what should Congress do when it reauthorizes the welfare law in 2002? First, lawmakers should not expect that most states would know what to do with funds earmarked for encouraging marriage or that their efforts are likely to be very successful. While there is nothing wrong with experimenting with marriage-education and counseling programs, so far there is little or no evidence to show that they will succeed. These programs are untested and don't tackle the real source of the problem, which is not a failure to marry but rather a failure to delay childbearing until marriage. Some people argue that we should aim marriage-counseling efforts at young cohabiting couples who have already had a baby. Maybe this will work. But it's a lot like trying to put the horse back in the barn. One hears a lot of talk about how we should support unwed fathers but not much about how to prevent them from becoming fathers in the first place.

For all these reasons, it would be better to provide states with flexible funding that could be used for a variety of efforts. This aid should be tied to success in achieving the basic purposes of the law, including its family-formation objectives. Based on existing research and experience, one of the most effective strategies states could choose if they want to reduce welfare dependency, child poverty, and the growth of single-parent families would be to emphasize programs that have a proven track record in reducing teen pregnancy. But let them choose from the full menu of approaches depending on their own assessment of the evidence and on local community values.

Finally, any diversion of resources from the more basic task of supporting needy families and "making work pay" would be unwise. Messages about marriage and about teen-pregnancy prevention need to target the younger generation. Those who are already single parents have little choice but to do the best job they can at making a living and raising their children, and they need our help.

> *"Washington has erected an impenetrable federal wall between parents and their minor children who receive prescription contraceptive drugs and devices from federally funded clinics."*

Teenagers Seeking Contraception Should Be Required to Notify Their Parents

Kevin Brady

Kevin Brady contends in the following viewpoint that parents should be informed if their children seek birth control from federally funded clinics. Under current law, these clinics are prohibited from notifying parents if their children request contraception. According to Brady, this statute puts teens at risk by preventing their parents from protecting them from sexual predators and potentially harmful contraceptives. Brady is a Republican representative from Texas.

As you read, consider the following questions:
1. According to the author, why does federal law prohibit clinics from notifying parents if their child seeks contraception?
2. What four federal programs, according to Brady, prevent clinics from releasing a minor's medical information?
3. What does the State's and Parental Rights Improvement Act stipulate, according to the author?

It is every parent's nightmare: Unbeknownst to you, your 12-year-old daughter secretly and repeatedly is being raped by her teacher. The teacher takes your child to a federally funded birth-control clinic to be injected with highly controversial contraceptives. His goal: to continue to assault her without fear of pregnancy.

Federal Requirements

Horrifying? It gets worse. Because the clinic is federally funded, its employees are not required to alert you. In fact, they can't. The federal government prohibits the clinic from telling parents their child is receiving prescription contraceptive drugs and devices. In this case, the clinic regularly is injecting your young daughter with Depo Provera, a powerful prescription contraceptive that increases the chances of developing breast cancer, blood clots and even strokes in young users.

The hormone is so powerful it has been used in some states to castrate convicted rapists. This time, however, the drug is not used on a rapist but by a rapist. The result: The teacher successfully hides the fact that he is preying on your daughter. The sexual assaults continue for the next year-and-a-half. Numerous shots are administered to your young daughter, who silently relents to an ever-increasing risk of dangerous side effects and emotional trauma.

Through it all, you know nothing. At her age the child is too scared to tell you. Believe it or not, the law of the land prevents you, the parent, from being told.

It sounds so disturbing it can't be true, can it? Sadly, it is. Real parents lived this nightmare in Illinois in 1997. And unbeknownst to most parents, this scene may be occurring all across America.

An Impenetrable Wall

One of America's more disturbing secrets is that Washington has erected an impenetrable federal wall between parents and their minor children who receive prescription contraceptive drugs and devices from federally funded clinics. It doesn't matter if your child is 9 years old or 16. It doesn't matter if she is receiving a surgically implanted intrauterine device

(IUD) or Norplant at age 13. Unbelievably, from the federal-government's standpoint you, the parent, must be kept in the dark. At a time in their young life when children need your help and guidance the most, Washington regulations block you from having a say in their health-care decisions.

The federal government doesn't believe you have earned the right to be informed. How can this happen? Well, some federal bureaucrat decided in the early 1970s that kids should be counted as "poor" as far as federal family-planning programs are concerned. Thus, by federal regulation, not law, clinics are required to keep it a secret when a teen-ager seeks contraceptive services.

Girls as young as 9 can and must be served by clinics distributing federally funded contraception. And, as we saw in Texas, if a state or a local community objects, too bad. Federal regulations trump state laws and parents have no say in the health decisions of their daughters even when those decisions can lead to increased risk of cancer, blood clots and strokes. That is outrageous.

Washington uses a heavy hand to enforce this wall of secrecy, quickly yanking funding from clinics that don't toe the line and threatening states that challenge their ironclad rules.

Ironically, states strive hard to protect young children from alcohol and drugs, from purchasing tobacco, getting a tattoo or driving a car at an early age. Schools require parental consent for field trips and suspend students who merely bring aspirin to school. Yet when the same states fight to ensure parents give their consent or at least be notified before their young daughter is injected with prescription contraceptives, Washington overrules them.

Fighting Back

Some states have rebelled. In 1997, the Texas Legislature passed a bill withholding state funds for family-planning programs unless parents were notified of any prescription drugs or devices administered to their minor children. As expected, Planned Parenthood [the world's largest reproductive health-care organization] sued, and a judge ruled in its favor. The court held the state of Texas could not limit the use of funds in this manner because the provision was in violation of four federal programs: Titles 10 (Family Planning), 19 (Medicaid), 20 (Social Services Block Grant) and Temporary Assistance to Needy Families. Later, the Texas Supreme Court wisely overturned the ruling—but only because of a technicality that Planned Parenthood had no standing to sue.

Strengthening Parental Rights

Although parental consent is required before a child can receive an aspirin at school, federally-funded Title X family planning clinics currently dispense contraceptives to teenagers (including prescription birth control pills and injections) without their parents' knowledge. Minors receive confidential services and are considered low-income and thereby eligible for free contraception—even though they are too young to legally consent to sex. Congress made major inroads by requiring these clinics to follow state statutory rape laws and report adults that prey on minors, but more needs to be done to help parents protect and guide their children.

Lee Terry, *Family First*, September 19, 2002.

The federal government wasted no time cracking down on the state, either. Under President Bill Clinton's health and human services secretary, Donna Shalala, the federal government threatened to withhold $93 million in federal funds if Texas didn't back off its parental-rights position.

As intended, Washington's heavy hand has had a chilling effect on other state legislatures considering similar common-sense efforts to protect minor children and ensure parental involvement in major medical decisions.

Restoring Parents' Rights

The federal government is wrong. Parents matter. For our children's sake, the rights of parents desperately need to be restored so they can be involved in these crucial medical decisions. Given the sacrifices that parents make for their children, the years instilling lifelong values and lessons and skills, the long nights nursing a sick or scared child, the daily trials and tribulations every parent faces as we work hard to give our children every opportunity to achieve their future dreams—parents have earned the right to be involved.

Parents will be expected to pick up the pieces when their

daughter contracts a sexually transmitted disease not prevented by many types of contraception and when she suffers the physical, let alone emotional, consequences of premarital sex. Yet the system is designed in such a way as to prevent parents from knowing what the government is doing to their children. Some will claim that there are teen-agers who can't talk to their parents, that not everyone has an "Ozzie-and-Harriet" type family. Perhaps. But it is a poor way to set public policy—keeping secrets from all parents because of troubles with a few.

States rights matter, too, as local legislators battle to protect their families from Washington decisions that weaken rather than strengthen families. Since Republicans took control of Congress, the U.S. House of Representatives has worked repeatedly to change these federal regulations. Unfortunately, the Senate has rejected each measure the House has sent its way, and President Clinton even threatened to veto the nation's health-care funding if the House-passed parental-notice provisions were not dropped.

Taking Action

To correct this problem, I again have introduced the State's and Parental Rights Improvement Act (HR 4783). This legislation says to the states that if you want to place thoughtful, commonsense safeguards on the distribution of prescription drugs to minors, the federal government can't interfere. It does not require parental notification before minors get prescription drugs, but merely allows it if a state enacts such safeguards. Passage of this legislation is needed to restore parental rights regarding their children's medical decisions and to return power to the states.

The beauty of my bill is that it allows states to decide for themselves how to set public policy in regard to parental involvement and prescription contraception drugs or devices.

Contrary to some people's claims, my bill does not mandate parental consent or parental notification on teen contraception. On the contrary, it simply says to states such as Texas that the federal government will not require parents be kept in the dark for their teens' health care.

Nor will the federal government tell a state how it should

handle teen-parent policy on contraceptive drugs or devices. My bill will allow a state to decide for itself, and allow that decision to be binding on the drugs and devices distributed to the state's teens.

If California wants to keep parents in the dark, it may. If Vermont wants minor girls to get injections of Depo Provera or surgically implanted Norplant, it may. I would hope that parents all across the nation would rally to get their state's legislature to restore their parental rights, but nothing in the bill requires this.

Lifting the Mandate of Secrecy

What this legislation ensures is the federal government will not be in a position to keep secrets from parents, especially in an area as important as their minor daughter's health. If the Texas Legislature wants to set a policy that parents must be notified before minor girls can receive contraceptive drugs and devices from Texas clinics and schools, it should be allowed. And under my bill, the federal regulatory mandate of secrecy is lifted.

Is the bill a panacea for parental rights? No. Is it a great first step toward restoring parental and state rights and long overdue? I believe it is.

If you asked the parents of that 12-year old girl, I think they'd tell you they agree with me—that Congress cannot act a moment too soon. It shouldn't take another federally funded nightmare.

Editor's note: The State's and Parental Rights Improvement Act was pending at the time of this publication.

"Access to contraceptive services is considered a fundamental privacy right."

Teenagers Seeking Contraception Should Not Be Required to Notify Their Parents

Center for Reproductive Law and Policy

In the following viewpoint, the Center for Reproductive Law and Policy (CRLP) argues that federal laws stipulating that teenagers do not need to notify their parents before they obtain birth control should be upheld. If teens are required to contact their parents when they seek condoms or birth control pills, many will be dissuaded from using contraception, putting them at risk for sexually transmitted diseases and unplanned pregnancies, according to the CRLP. Moreover, the organization contends, some teens risk angry or violent reactions from their parents, who may disapprove of their sexual activity. The CRLP is a nonprofit legal advocacy organization dedicated to promoting and defending women's reproductive rights.

As you read, consider the following questions:
1. What are two examples offered by the CRLP of minors who would face harm if they were required to notify their parents that they needed birth control?
2. Which two federal programs require federally funded clinics to maintain teens' confidentiality, according to the CRLP?
3. Why does the organization contend that parental consent for contraception is unconstitutional?

I ncreasingly, proposals are being introduced to restrict teens' access to reproductive health care by calling for parental consent or notification. Currently, no state or federal laws require minors to get parental consent in order to get contraception.

Examples of Minors Who Would Face Harm

Teens in a variety of circumstances would be affected if required to obtain parental consent for contraception:

- A young woman seeking contraception from a clinic—birth control pills, DepoProvera, diaphragm—would be forced to obtain parental permission
- A minor who buys condoms at a pharmacy could be turned away without parental consent
- A teen who seeks emergency contraception because of forced or unanticipated intercourse would need approval, even though emergency contraception must be used within 72 hours of unprotected intercourse.

Two types of mandatory parental contact for contraception are sometimes proposed:

- Mandatory parental consent would force teenagers to get permission from one or two parents before getting contraception.
- Mandatory parental notification would require young people to tell one or two parents about their plans to get contraception. Mandatory notification poses the same danger of discouraging contraceptive use by teens as does the requirement of consent. If a minor is fearful about discussing contraception with a parent, there is no difference between 'telling' the parent and getting parental permission.

Federal Programs Require Confidentiality for Teens

Two federal programs—Title X and Medicaid—protect teens' privacy and prohibit parental consent requirements for teens seeking contraception. Title X provides funds to states for family planning services; Medicaid covers health care services for low-income women. Both programs mandate that, in exchange for receiving monies from the federal government, health care services treat all patients confidentially, including teens.

Attempts by states to implement parental consent requirements for contraceptive services that are funded by these programs have been invalidated when challenged in court. Courts find that the requirements impermissibly conflict with federal program requirements. Federal program rules mandating confidentiality preempt state efforts to make new requirements.

Both Consent and Notification Damage Teens

Parental contact requirements discourage teens from seeking contraception, even though they may already be sexually active. Confidentiality can be a determining factor for teens deciding whether or not to seek contraceptive protection.

Teenagers Need Access to Contraceptive Services

More than half the women in the United States have intercourse before their 17th birthday. While the teen pregnancy rate today has dropped slightly in the past twenty years, almost one million teens become pregnant each year. A sexually active teen using no contraception has a 90% chance of becoming pregnant within a one year period, according to the Alan Guttmacher Institute.

Lack of contraception increases the chances of unintended pregnancy. Nearly 80% of teen pregnancies are unplanned in the U.S. Teen pregnancy rates are much higher in the U.S. than in other industrial countries—double the rates in England; nine times as high as the Netherlands. Lack of contraception also increases the possibility of exposure to sexually transmitted diseases. About three million U.S. teens acquire a sexually transmitted infection every year.

Parental Contact Laws Threaten Teens' Health

Supporters of measures forcing teens to notify or get consent from their parents argue that they promote the best interests of young women and improve family communications.

These arguments are out of touch with reality. These proposed laws threaten adolescent health and well-being. Even teens who could comply with parental consent requirements will face delays in getting contraceptive services. Additional clinic visits, missed school or work time, and increased expense will result.

Many young women live in nontraditional situations—with one parent, a stepparent, other relatives, or on their own. Contact with biological parents, if required by law, may be impossible.

Same Activity, Less Protection

Requirements that teenagers notify their parents or get their consent before obtaining contraception endanger the public health and violate the law. Coercing parental involvement in teenagers' decisions regarding contraception would not decrease teenage sexual activity, but would instead lead an increasing number of teens to forego protection when they have sex. As rates of unprotected sex climb, so does the incidence of unintended pregnancy, teenage childbearing, abortion, and sexually transmitted disease. Nor would parental involvement requirements create by fiat families in which open communication is both safe and constructive. Moreover, conditioning a teenager's access to contraception on parental consent or notification is unconstitutional, as well as contrary to the confidentiality mandates of certain federal statutes.

American Civil Liberties Union, "ACLU Opposes Parental Involvement Requirements for Teenagers Seeking Contraceptives," April 1, 1999.

Some teens face violence or other severe consequences from parents as a result of informing their parents that they are seeking contraceptive services. Minors fearful of retribution may forgo using contraception altogether, even though they are already sexually active.

Teens who seek contraceptive services are generally sexually active already. They benefit from meeting with health care providers, who can provide screening, counseling about sexually transmitted diseases, and education about other reproductive health concerns.

States May Not Impose Additional Restrictions on Title X Programs

Several courts have found that state parental consent requirements may not be imposed on federally funded family planning programs. Where states accept Title X and Medicaid funds, they cannot require minors to obtain parental consent prior to using those services.

Parental Consent for Contraception Is Unconstitutional

Minors have a right to privacy that includes their ability to use contraception.

The U.S. Supreme Court said in 1977 that denial of contraception is not a permissible way to deter sexual activity.

Although states may require parental consent for a minor's abortion when sufficient alternatives, such as judicial bypass, are in place, the same reasoning does not apply to contraception. According to the U.S. Supreme Court, "The states' interest in protection of the mental and physical health of the pregnant minor, and in protection of potential life are clearly more implicated by the abortion decision than by the decision to use a nonhazardous contraceptive."

Access to contraceptive services is considered a fundamental privacy right and has remained so for over three decades.

Endangering Teens' Lives

Placing barriers on teen access to contraception is dangerous to the health and welfare of young women because it increases their risk of unplanned pregnancies. The costs to society from teen pregnancy are enormous.

While programs with federal family planning money are forbidden from requiring parental consent or notice for teen services, teens also have a constitutional right to privacy that encompasses their decision to obtain contraception, a right that lawmakers should acknowledge and respect.

Periodical Bibliography

The following articles have been selected to supplement the diverse views presented in this chapter.

Sue Alford	"What's Wrong with Federal Abstinence-Only-Until-Marriage Requirements?" *Transitions*, March 2001.
Jacqueline Corcoran	"Preventing Adolescent Pregnancy: A Review of Programs and Practices," *Social Work*, January 2000.
Patricia Donovan	"Can Statutory Rape Laws Be Effective in Preventing Adolescent Pregnancy?" *Family Planning Perspectives*, January/February 1997.
Carol Ford	"Preventing Teen Pregnancy with Emergency Contraception: An Opportunity We Should Not Be Missing," *Archives of Pediatrics & Adolescent Medicine*, August 1998.
Donna Futterman	"Do Abstinence-Only Sex Education Programs Work?" *Family Practice News*, July 15, 2000.
Russell W. Gough	"The Hunt for the Sex-Education Truth," *World & I*, August 1997.
Alison Hadley	"How to Cut Teenage Pregnancies," *New Statesman*, July 3, 1998.
Debra W. Haffner	"What's Wrong with Abstinence-Only Sexuality Education Programs?" *SIECUS*, 1997.
Tamara Kreinin	"Keep Kids From Making Babies," *NEA Today*, November 1998.
Jodie Morse and Hillary Hylton	"Preaching Chastity in the Classroom," *Time*, October 18, 1999.
Sheron C. Patterson	"Churches Need to Teach Teens About Sex," *Dallas Morning News*, September 23, 2000.
Annys Shin	"OK, Boys and Girls—Don't Do It!" *National Journal*, October 25, 1997.
Gary Thomas	"True Love Waits," *Christianity Today*, March 1, 1999.
Paul V. Trad	"Assessing the Patterns That Prevent Teenage Pregnancy," *Adolescence*, Spring 1999.

CHAPTER 3

How Can Society Deal with Teenage Crime and Violence?

Chapter Preface

In 1997 fourteen-year-old Michael Carneal fired a .22 caliber handgun at an informal prayer group in his high school in West Paducah, Kentucky, killing three students and wounding five. In Pearl, Mississippi, sixteen-year-old Luke Woodham first killed his mother and then went to school and shot nine students, killing two, in 1998. In the same year, fifteen-year-old Kip Kinkel shot and killed his parents and two classmates and wounded twenty-three others.

School shootings such as these provide disturbing evidence of an increase in gun violence among teenagers. Between 1979 and 1999, gunfire killed more than eighty-seven thousand children and teens in the United States. According to the Justice Department, between 1986 and 1992, the total number of juveniles killed by firearms rose by 144 percent. Gun killings by teenagers rose from five thousand in 1980 to more than seventy-five thousand in 1997. Common Sense about Kids and Guns, a gun violence prevention organization, contends that teen suicide by firearm increased 21 percent from 1998 to 2000. Many people argue that easy access to guns in the home and lax laws regarding the sale of guns contribute to increased firearm violence among youth.

According to Sue Peschin, a spokesperson for the Consumer Federation of America, "School shootings often involve guns found in the home." The United States Secret Service National Threat Assessment Center claims that two-thirds of the forty-one students involved in thirty-seven school shooting incidents since 1974 got their guns from their own home or the home of a relative. A 1998 study by the Center to Prevent Handgun Violence (CPHV) found that more than 40 percent of American homes with children also contain guns; in 25 percent of those homes, guns are kept loaded and unlocked. Victoria Reggie Kennedy, president of Common Sense about Kids and Guns, argues that recent school shootings demonstrate the "overwhelming importance of adult responsibility to ensure that no child or teen ever encounters a loaded or improperly stored firearm in the home." She suggests that gun owners always keep their guns unloaded, locked, and stored out of reach of children and teens.

Others argue that the best way to protect young people from gun violence is to reduce the number of guns in society. The Coalition to Stop Gun Violence estimates that there are 192 million guns in private hands. Activists contend that the government should enact legislation that tightens restrictions on purchasing guns, especially at gun shows. Every year, an estimated two thousand to five thousand gun shows take place across the nation. In most states it is legal for private collectors to sell their guns without a waiting period or background check on the purchaser. The federal Gun Show Accountability Act of 1999 was designed to close the loophole that allows private gun collectors to sell guns without investigation into the buyer. The act is currently being reviewed by a legislative committee.

According to Sarah Brady, head of the CPHV, "Whether a gun is taken from the home or purchased at a gun show or on the streets, it is simply far too easy for young people to get a hold of firearms in this country." She and others maintain that gun owners must ensure that their guns are safely out of reach of kids and teens, and they urge lawmakers to pass legislation reducing the number of guns in society. Only time will tell whether these efforts to reduce gun violence among teens will be successful. Authors in the following chapter debate other ways to reduce teen crime and violence, such as curfews and zero tolerance laws.

> "If a juvenile is accused of murdering, raping or assaulting someone with a deadly weapon, the suspect should automatically be sent to adult criminal court."

More Teenage Criminals Should Be Tried as Adults

Linda J. Collier

In the following viewpoint, Linda J. Collier contends that teenagers who knowingly commit adult crimes should face adult punishment. She maintains that recent acts of violence, such as school shootings in Paducah, Kentucky, and Jonesboro, Arkansas, illustrate that the incidence of violent crime committed by teens is rising. Unfortunately, she asserts, the juvenile justice system is not equipped to deal with the increasing number of violent teenage offenders and should be overhauled. Collier, an attorney in Pennsylvania, has worked in the juvenile courts.

As you read, consider the following questions:
1. What is the difference between crimes committed by juveniles today and crimes committed by juveniles more than twenty years ago, as stated by the author?
2. How does Collier define a guardian ad litem?
3. According to the author, why are state laws regarding waivers to adult court inconsistent?

When prosecutor Brent Davis said he wasn't sure if he could charge 11-year-old Andrew Golden and 13-year-old Mitchell Johnson as adults after March 24, 1998's, slaughter in Jonesboro, Arkansas, I cringed. But not for the reasons you might think.

Children First, Criminals Second

I knew he was formulating a judgment based on laws that have not had a major overhaul for more than 100 years. I knew his hands were tied by the longstanding creed that juvenile offenders, generally defined as those under the age of 18, are to be treated rather than punished. I knew he would have to do legal cartwheels to get the case out of the juvenile system. But most of all, I cringed because today's juvenile suspects—even those who are accused of committing the most violent crimes—are still regarded by the law as children first and criminals second.

As astonishing as the Jonesboro events were, this is hardly the first time that children with access to guns and other weapons have brought tragedy to a school. Only weeks before the Jonesboro shootings, three girls in Paducah, Kentucky, were killed in their school lobby when a 14-year-old classmate allegedly opened fire on them. Authorities said he had several guns with him, and the alleged murder weapon was one of seven stolen from a neighbor's garage. And the day after the Jonesboro shootings, a 14-year-old in Daly City, California, was charged as a juvenile after he allegedly fired at his middle-school principal with a semiautomatic handgun.

It's not a new or unusual phenomenon for children to commit violent crimes at younger and younger ages, but it often takes a shocking incident to draw our attention to a trend already in progress. According to the U.S. Department of Justice, crimes committed by juveniles increased by 60 percent from 1984 to 1998. Where juvenile delinquency was once limited to truancy or vandalism, juveniles now are more likely to be the perpetrators of serious and deadly crimes such as arson, aggravated assault, rape and murder. And these violent offenders increasingly include those as young as the Jonesboro suspects. Since 1965, the number of 12-year-olds arrested for violent crimes has doubled and the number of 13- and 14-year-olds has tripled, according to government statistics.

Those statistics are a major reason why we need to revamp our antiquated juvenile justice system. Nearly every state, including Arkansas, has laws that send most youthful violent offenders to the juvenile courts, where they can only be found "delinquent" and confined in a juvenile facility (typically not past age 21). In recent years, many states have enacted changes in their juvenile crime laws, and some have lowered the age at which a juvenile can be tried as an adult for certain violent crimes. Virginia, for example, has reduced its minimum age to 14, and suspects accused of murder and aggravated malicious wounding are automatically waived to adult court. Illinois is now sending some 13-year-olds to adult court after a hearing in juvenile court. In Kansas, a 1996 law allows juveniles as young as 10 to be prosecuted as adults in some cases. These are steps in the right direction, but too many states still treat violent offenders under 16 as juveniles who belong in the juvenile system.

Failing to Treat and Punish

My views are not those of a frustrated prosecutor. I have represented children as a court-appointed guardian ad litem, or temporary guardian, in the Philadelphia juvenile justice system. Loosely defined, a guardian ad litem is responsible for looking after the best interest of a neglected or rebellious child who has come into the juvenile courts. It is often a humbling experience as I try to help children whose lives have gone awry, sometimes because of circumstances beyond their control.

My experience has made me believe that the system is doing a poor job at treatment as well as punishment. One of my "girls," a chronic truant, was a foster child who longed to be adopted. She often talked of how she wanted a pink room, a frilly bunk bed and sisters with whom she could share her dreams. She languished in foster care from ages 2 to 13 because her drug-ravaged mother would not relinquish her parental rights. Initially, the girl refused to tolerate the half-life that the state had maintained was in her best interest. But as it became clear that we would never convince her mother to give up her rights, the girl became a frequent run-away. Eventually she ended up pregnant, wandering from place to place and committing adult crimes to survive. No longer a child, not quite a woman, she is the kind of teenager offender for whom the juvenile system has little or nothing to offer.

Adult Crime, Adult Punishment

The simple fact is that fully competent and mature juveniles are fully capable of committing the same crime as a competent adult. The results of the crime are the same. In burglary, an innocent person was robbed of his possessions. In murder, an innocent person was robbed of his life. As Katrina Ng, Santa Clara University freshman answered, "If they commit the adult crimes, they should pay the adult consequences. It's not as if they don't know the difference between right and wrong."

And even in the extreme cases where right and wrong were indistinguishable to the immature juvenile, the adult justice system would be better equipped to prosecute him, allowing for mitigating circumstances and giving due process. This way, justice is best achieved—on both sides.

Hanna Chiou, *Digital High*, 2000.

A brief history: Proceedings in juvenile justice began in 1890 in Chicago, where the original mandate was to save wayward children and protect them from the ravages of society. The system called for children to be processed through an appendage of the family court. By design, juveniles were to be kept away from the court's criminal side, the district attorney and adult correctional institutions.

Typically, initial procedures are informal, non-threatening and not open to public scrutiny. A juvenile suspect is interviewed by an "intake" officer who determines the child's fate. The intake officer may issue a warning, lecture and release; he may detain the suspect; or, he may decide to file a petition, subjecting the child to juvenile "adjudication" proceedings. If the law allows, the intake officer may make a recommendation that the juvenile be transferred to adult criminal court.

An adjudication is similar to a hearing, rather than a trial, although the juvenile may be represented by counsel and a juvenile prosecutor will represent the interests of the community. It is important to note that throughout the proceedings, no matter which side of the fence the parties are on, the operating principle is that everyone is working in the best interests of the child. Juvenile court judges do not issue findings of guilt, but decide whether a child is delinquent. If delinquency is found, the judge must decide the child's fate. Should the child be sent back to the family—assuming there is one? Declare him or her "in need of supervision," which brings in the intense help of social services? Remove the child from the family and place him or her in foster care? Confine the child to a state institution for juvenile offenders?

This system was developed with truants, vandals and petty thieves in mind. But this model is not appropriate for the violent juvenile offender of today. Detaining a rapist or murderer in a juvenile facility until the age of 18 or 21 isn't even a slap on the hand. If a juvenile is accused of murdering, raping or assaulting someone with a deadly weapon, the suspect should automatically be sent to adult criminal court. What's to ponder?

Overhauling Juvenile Justice Laws

With violent crime becoming more prevalent among the junior set, it's a mystery why there hasn't been a major overhaul of juvenile justice laws long before now. Will the Jonesboro shootings be the incident that makes us take a hard look at the current system? When it became evident that the early release of Jesse Timmendequas—whose murder of 7-year-old Megan Kanka in New Jersey sparked national outrage—had caused unwarranted tragedy, legislative action was swift. Now New Jersey has Megan's Law, which requires the advance notification of a sexual predator's release into a neighborhood. Other states have followed suit.

It is unequivocally clear that the same type of mandate is needed to establish a uniform minimum age for trying juveniles as adults. As it stands now, there is no consistency in state laws governing waivers to adult court. One reason for this lack of uniformity is the absence of direction from the federal government or Congress. The Bureau of Justice Statistics reports that adjacent states such as New York and Pennsylvania respond differently to 16-year-old criminals, with New York tending to treat offenders of that age as adults and Pennsylvania handling them in the juvenile justice system.

Federal prosecution of juveniles is not totally unheard of, but it is uncommon. The Bureau of Justice Statistics estimates that during 1994, at least 65 juveniles were referred to the attorney general for transfer to adult status. In such cases, the U.S. attorney's office must certify a substantial federal interest in the case and show that one of the following is true: The state does not have jurisdiction; the state refuses to assume jurisdiction or the state does not have adequate services for juvenile offenders; the offense is a violent felony, drug trafficking or firearm offense as defined by the U.S. Code.

Exacting hurdles, but not insurmountable. In the Jonesboro case, prosecutor Davis has been exploring ways to enlist the federal court's jurisdiction. [Andrew Golden and Mitchell Johnson were sentenced in juvenile court.] Whatever happens, federal prosecutions of young offenders are clearly not the long-term answer. The states must act. So as far as I can see, the next step is clear: Children who knowingly engage in adult conduct and adult crimes should automatically be subject to adult rules and adult prison time.

*"Subjecting youths to [adult punishment]
. . . undermines the very values of a society
that insists that the punishment fit the
crime."*

Teenage Criminals Should Not Be Tried as Adults

Lise A. Young

Lise A. Young, a juvenile dependency lawyer, contends that trying teenage criminals as adults is unfair. She argues that youthful offenders are not as cognitively developed or mature as adults and, therefore, should not be held accountable for their crimes in the same way that adults are. She maintains that alternative treatment programs, such as community courts and restorative justice programs, are more effective at rehabilitating juvenile criminals than adult sentences.

As you read, consider the following questions:

1. According to the author, who initiated juvenile courts and why?
2. What are three reasons why adult sentencing for minors is immoral, as stated by Young?
3. According to Young, what are restorative justice programs?

Lise A. Young, "Suffer the Children: The Basic Principle of Juvenile Justice Is to Treat the Child, Not Punish the Offense," *America*, vol. 185, October 22, 2001, pp. 19–26. Copyright © 2001 by America Press, Inc., 106 West 56th Street, New York, NY 10019, www.americamagazine.org. Reproduced by permission.

There is growing public pressure to charge, try, convict and sentence juvenile offenders in adult criminal courts. This is a misguided and simplistic approach to a complex problem. Proven constructive alternatives exist that can be implemented if the public and its leaders are committed to real reform of America's juvenile justice system.

The Genesis and Operation of Juvenile Courts

Juvenile courts are the product of a 19th-century reform movement that sought to address the rising number of poor and homeless children and the potential they created for increased juvenile crime in post-Industrial Revolution America. Contrary to popular belief, liberal social reformers were not the main supporters of this movement: police and prosecutors were instrumental in advocating separate juvenile courts, because youths tried in adult courts were so often released or found innocent due to jurors' sympathy. In fact, Illinois, the first state to enact legislation establishing a separate juvenile court system, did so as the result of a state supreme court decision that had held it unlawful for judges to institutionalize children for noncriminal behavior.

From their inception, juvenile courts had a very different purpose from that of adult courts. The goal of juvenile courts was and is to try to reintegrate young offenders into the greater social fabric through the use of highly individualized sentences (called dispositions), whereas the purpose of adult criminal courts was and is primarily to punish. Juvenile courts have very broad discretion to order a wide range of interventions. A young offender can be returned home to his or her family with no services, returned home on informal probation with a commitment by the young offender and/or family to voluntarily participate in various designated services, returned home on formal probation subject to completing mandatory services designated by the court, detained (held in temporary custody by law enforcement, then released to foster care in a structured plan of services) or incarcerated. Incarceration in such circumstances is usually in a juvenile detention facility, although some states are increasingly inclined to send serious juvenile offenders to adult prisons. The key consideration in juvenile court disposition lies in determining what factors caused a youth to go astray, and then ordering whatever interventions the judge—with input from the prosecutor and/or probation officer, child welfare professionals, family members and defense counsel—deems necessary to prevent further criminality. Thus, even incarceration is viewed primarily as a corrective, not a punitive, measure.

Behind this goal lies a fundamental principle of Anglo-American jurisprudence: punishment should be proportionate to the level of evil intent (mens rea) behind a crime. Because children and adolescents are not fully developed cognitively, morally and emotionally, they should not be held to the same standards of moral accountability, but rather should be held accountable in a developmentally appropriate way.

But in the last 10 years, juvenile courts have been criticized for being too lenient and incapable of dealing with the so-called "super-predators," who commit very few, but sensationally publicized, crimes. Juvenile courts, these critics say, were not designed to handle such crimes effectively and are unable to do so. They argue that public safety demands certain and more severe punishment of serious juvenile offenders, and that a system in which 73 percent of all referrals end with no formal services or sanctions whatsoever is flawed. They claim further that the rehabilitative goal of juvenile courts is unrealistic, given the high cost and broad range of services needed to salvage young offenders. These tough-on-crime voices have been heard by legislatures in nearly all 50 states, which over the last 10 years have modified their laws to allow more youths to be tried as adults, to reduce the informality and confidentiality of juvenile court proceedings and to increase the severity of punishments. In 2000, for example, California voters approved by 62 percent a voter initiative measure—Proposition 21—that incorporated provisions like these.

Adult Crime, Adult Time

Many tough-on-crime advocates call for certain crimes to be automatically heard in adult criminal courts, with convicted offenders subject to sentencing under adult standards. Such proposals focus on the gravity of the act and its immediate impact on the victim and society, rather than on the inner disposition and motivations of the youthful perpetrator. Although intention still plays some role in determining the severity of the crime, considerations of the juvenile's immature judgment, dysfunctional family life, low cognitive function, poor impulse control and other factors relating directly to the minor's inner disposition are deemed irrelevant. In such an approach, minors are presumed to have the same ability to comprehend the nature of their act, to freely consent to committing it and to be totally invested in committing it as an adult—simply by virtue of the gravity of the act itself and the severity of its impact on the victim.

A graphic example of this approach was a Michigan case involving a 14-year-old boy with an I.Q. of 74 (borderline deficient) who hit a classmate and took his $2 lunch money. The boy was charged as an adult for the crime. The prosecutor said in defense of his decision: "The gravity of the crime is not diminished by whatever learning disabilities the perpetrator may have. The victim was no less frightened or traumatized."

The principle of proportionality provides a framework for evaluating the morality of sentencing juveniles as adults. That principle states that three factors must be evaluated in determining a moral course of action: (1) the means used will not cause more harm than necessary to achieve the value; (2) there is no less harmful way at present to protect the value; and (3) the means used to achieve the value will not undermine it.

Racial Disparities

Examined in the light of this three-factor test, sentencing and punishing children by the adult criminal standards in use in this country is flagrantly immoral. First, the impact of sentencing juveniles in adult courts falls disproportionately on minority youth. Nonwhite youths in California, for example, are more than eight times more likely than white youths to be sentenced by an adult court to incarceration in a youth facility and three times more likely to be transferred to adult court for trial and sentencing. This violates the third criterion above by seriously undermining the credibility of the juvenile justice system. How can a system of law that results in such gross disparities among the races be considered fair and equitable?

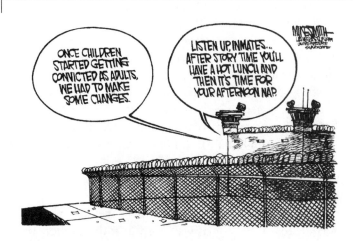

Smith. © 1999 by *Las Vegas Sun*. Reprinted by permission of United Feature Syndicate.

Second, sentencing young people to adult punishments subjects youthful offenders to conditions that are unacceptable for children. Adult prisons offer virtually no counseling and little or no education at the secondary level. For such youths, long sentences served in adult prisons basically end all possibilities for a meaningful life once they are released as adults. Additionally, youths incarcerated in adult facilities are many times more likely to be sexually assaulted, beaten by staff or attacked with a weapon. Youth-only facilities for serious juvenile offenders convicted in adult courts often are no better. A Michigan youth prison's rate of critical incidents (from assaults to attempted suicides) was almost three times that of the state's adult maximum security prison. Subjecting youths to this sort of abuse is surely not only disproportionate to their moral culpability, but also undermines the very values of a society that insists that the punishment fit the crime.

Nor is the practice of sentencing and incarcerating juveniles as if they were adults acceptable according to established Catholic moral teachings on crime and punishment. According to the Catechism of the Catholic Church, there are three justifications for punishment: rehabilitation of the criminal, deterrence and retribution/preservation of public order (No. 2266). Clearly, incarcerating juvenile offenders in facilities that effectively end their chances for a productive life are anything but rehabilitative. There is little or no proof that stiff sentences for juvenile offenders are a deterrent to similar offenses, either by other juveniles or the same juvenile; in fact, statistical studies to date suggest just the opposite. A study done in Connecticut in 1996 concluded that young offenders sentenced to alternative programs have a significantly lower rate of rearrest than juveniles sentenced to adult correctional facilities. This finding was adopted by the California Legislative Analyst's office in its analysis of the probable impacts of Proposition 21, the youth crime initiative mentioned above. A Florida study likewise showed that the recidivism [rearrest] rate among juveniles who were transferred to adult court was significantly higher than among juveniles who had been tried and sentenced in juvenile courts; and a New York study confirmed the Connecticut finding that the rearrest rate for children sentenced in juvenile court was 29 percent lower than for juveniles sentenced in adult criminal courts.

Willful ignorance is evident in certain public perceptions of the so-called juvenile crime "epidemic." For example, 60 percent of the respondents in a California poll felt that youths committed "most crime nowadays," when in fact 80 percent of the arrests in 1996 were of adult offenders. Adults committed 10 times as many homicides in 1999 as juveniles. Seventy-one percent of respondents in a national 1999 poll thought it was likely a school shooting would happen in their community, even though the chance of that actually happening was less than 1 in 2,000,000! In fact, in 1998, youth crime was at its lowest rate in the 25-year history of the U.S. Census Bureau's polling data on youth crime. Youth homicides alone were down 68 percent since their peak in 1993. And yet, although youth crime is down, public outrage is up. People are choosing either not to hear at all or to hear only the information that supports their irrational fears and prejudices.

A Proposal for Action

There are alternatives to the unjust measures that have been, and continue to be, legislated to deal with the problem of youthful offenders. Legislators should resist the temptation to "simplify" matters by eliminating juvenile courts entirely, because such tactics are both immoral and ineffective. Instead, the basic principle of juvenile justice—to treat the child, not punish the offense—needs to be furthered in constructive new ways.

First, there should be increased efforts to identify and provide services to at-risk youths before they commit crimes. Such youths are not all that difficult to identify. They are frequently from dysfunctional families with issues of domestic violence, substance abuse, physical and/or sexual abuse; they are often truants; and they tend to resort to violence as a means of settling conflict. Such youths and their families need to be directed into publicly funded programs that can provide them with new and better educational and coping skills (e.g., tutoring, mentoring, cash incentives for graduation, conflict resolution programs in the school, parenting instruction and youth employment programs). Critics may argue that an approach of this kind is too expensive, but statistics prove that in the long run, prevention is cheaper than punishment. California, for example, recently showed renewed commitment to a rational juvenile justice policy when it paired $121 million in preventive program funding with the same amount in prosecutorial and law enforcement funding—the largest amount ever dedicated there in a single year to youth crime prevention.

Second, once juveniles are caught in the justice system, it is critical to target first-time offenders for special intervention. One program in Orange County, California, which targets first-time offenders for intensive services, achieved almost a 30 percent reduction in the number of probation violations or additional charges filed against young first-time offenders: a rate of repeat offenses less than half of the control group's, and an incarceration rate about a third that of nonparticipants.

Finally, innovative alternatives to the criminal justice/punishment model, which have already been developed, should be gradually integrated into the system—especially where nonviolent crimes are involved. Such innovative alternatives include restorative justice programs and community courts. The former (which have been implemented effectively in Australia, New Zealand and at least one county in the state of Oregon), provide for carefully structured meetings among offenders, victims, their families and other community members in which the offender is confronted personally with the wrong that his/her conduct has caused others, and is involved directly in devising a way to repair the damage or harm he or she has caused. Statistical studies to date suggest that there are lower recidivism rates and greater satisfaction among participants in restorative justice projects than among those involved in traditional punishment-driven programs. Community court programs offer another alternative to traditional juvenile or adult court systems: there, juvenile offenders give back to the community they have harmed, either through money, service or both, instead of doing time in conventional correctional facilities.

I participate in programs that offer mediation as an alternative to litigation, and have seen alternative dispute resolution successfully implemented schoolwide among junior high staff, teachers and students. Our local court has had a VOMP (Victim-Offender Mediation Project) for juvenile offenders in place on an experimental basis for the last two years. The experience of owning one's anger and working through conflict to resolution with an opponent, rather than seeking revenge, can be truly transformative. I have also lobbied for implementation of such programs at other levels of our local court system and at our parish school. Parents, educators and especially religious leaders should work toward instituting conflict resolution and conflict management programs like these in their schools and should encourage the use of such alternative dispute resolution methods in place of traditional confrontational approaches in their workplaces too. It is important to counter the massive disinformation that the popular press is currently disseminating about juvenile crime and justice issues. It is also critical for us to learn to practice, and for our children to grow up with, models of dispute resolution other than the adversarial methods we are used to.

> "For over a century, communities in the
> United States have imposed juvenile
> curfews to help maintain order and reduce
> crime committed by youths."

Curfew Laws Can Reduce Teenage Crime and Violence

J. Richard Ward Jr.

In the following viewpoint, J. Richard Ward Jr. argues that youth curfew laws can help prevent teenage crime and violence by reducing teens' exposure to drug abuse and gangs. He describes a successful curfew program in Charlottesville, Virginia, to illustrate how curfews not only protect the community from teen criminals but also protect teens from the more unsavory elements in the community. According to Ward, the project found that three main factors are essential to a successful curfew program: community acceptance, consistent enforcement practices, and accurate record keeping. Ward is a contributor to the *FBI Law Enforcement Bulletin*.

As you read, consider the following questions:
1. According to the author, when did curfews first appear and why?
2. What prompted the Charlottesville City Council to enact youth curfew laws, as stated by Ward?
3. According to Ward, what were three benefits to implementing youth curfew laws in Charlottesville, Virginia?

J. Richard Ward Jr., "Implementing Juvenile Curfew Programs," *FBI Law Enforcement Bulletin*, vol. 69, March 2000, pp. 15–17. Copyright © 2000 by *FBI Law Enforcement Bulletin*. Reproduced by permission.

B esides meaning "the sounding of a bell at evening," the word curfew also denotes "a regulation enjoining the withdrawal of usually specified persons (as juveniles or military personnel) from the streets or the closing of business establishments or places of assembly at a stated hour" [according to Webster's Collegiate Dictionary]. The latter application has begun to appear ever increasingly in research studies and articles as a way to stem juvenile crime and victimization.

For over a century, American communities have imposed curfews at various times in an effort to maintain social order. For example, curfews first appeared during the 1890s in large urban areas to decrease crime among immigrant youth. During World War II, many communities again turned to curfews as a method of control for parents busily engaged in the war effort. More recent interest in curfews occurred as a response to the increase in juvenile crime and gang activity during the 1970s.

Today, lawmakers, government leaders, social scientists, and law enforcement authorities have begun to examine the legalities, planning, effects, and benefits of juvenile curfews. Most believe that any law that may decrease the number of juveniles involved in illegal activities and possibly reduce the crimes perpetrated against juveniles would benefit their communities. Although critics have voiced concerns about infringing on the rights of juveniles and their parents, as well as the effectiveness of curfews on crime rates, many communities have found curfews beneficial.

The Charlottesville Experience

Located about 70 miles northwest of Richmond in the foothills of the Blue Ridge Mountains, Charlottesville, Virginia, encompasses over 10 square miles and has a population of nearly 40,000 residents. Although the community had experienced relatively little juvenile violence, the city decided to adopt a curfew more as a preventive measure to protect its children from harmful influences, such as drug abuse and gang involvement, and to promote healthy behavior, rather than as a response to an increase in juvenile crime. Complaints of young people riding bicycles or loitering on the streets at 1 or 2 o'clock in the morning prompted the city council, the police department, and concerned community members to find a way not only to protect these youngsters but also to help parents enforce their own curfew rules.

After several months of study and deliberation, the Charlottesville City Council enacted a juvenile curfew on December 16, 1996. The city council designed the curfew ordinance—

• to promote the general welfare and protect the general public through the reduction of juvenile violence and crime within the city;

• to promote the safety and well-being of the city's youngest citizens, persons under the age of 17, whose inexperience renders them particularly vulnerable to becoming participants in unlawful activities, especially unlawful drug activities, and to being victimized by older perpetrators of crime; and

• to foster and strengthen parental responsibility for children.

With these basic tenets in mind, the Charlottesville Police Department examined other communities with positive curfew experiences and learned the importance of the three main factors that go into making successful curfew programs: community acceptance, consistent enforcement practices, and accurate record keeping.

Community Acceptance

First and foremost, community members must accept the curfew. Parents and guardians must realize that they will have to assist in its enforcement on the family level and always know the whereabouts of their children after curfew hours. Law enforcement authorities alone cannot effectively enforce curfews, all adults concerned with the safety of their community's children must join in the effort. For example, one way that the Charlottesville Police Department gained community support for the curfew involved using its school resource officers to inform all school personnel and students. This allowed students to learn firsthand about the curfew and its impact on them.

Additionally, communities should implement comprehensive curfew programs that change the punitive nature of the curfew into an intervention process that can attack the primary causes of juvenile delinquency and victimization. These programs should include such strategies as—

• creating a dedicated curfew center or using recreation centers and churches to house curfew violators;

• staffing these centers with social service professionals and community volunteers;

• offering referrals to social service providers and counseling classes for juvenile violators and their families;

• establishing procedures—such as fines, counseling, or community service—for repeat offenders;

• developing recreation, employment, antidrug, and antigang programs; and

• providing hot lines for follow-up services and crisis intervention.

These strategies proved beneficial in Charlottesville,

A Two-Part Goal

The stated goal of most curfew laws is twofold: to prevent juvenile crime and to protect youth from victimization. According to researchers William Ruefle's and Kenneth Mike Reynolds's analysis, those who support juvenile curfews indicate that neighborhoods afflicted with high rates of crime may use curfews as a "means to protect nondelinquent youth from crime and to deny delinquent youth the opportunity to engage in criminal behavior." By keeping youth under the age of 18 off the street, curfews are expected to reduce the incidence of crime among the cohort most likely to offend, according to the Federal Bureau of Investigation's (FBI's) 1994 Uniform Crime Report (UCR). Since juvenile perpetrators of crime often take as their victims other youth, it is hoped that rates of youth victimization will drop as well.

Curfews are credited by some with restoring and maintaining order in lower crime neighborhoods, according to the Ruefle and Reynolds analysis. In addition to equipping law enforcement with tools to keep youth off the streets, curfews provide parents with a legitimate, legal basis for restricting the activities of their children. It is easier for parents to place boundaries on their children's activities, proponents argue, when other youth in the neighborhood are similarly restricted by a specific time to return home.

Office of Juvenile Justice and Delinquency Prevention, *Juvenile Justice Reform Initiatives in the States: 1994–1996*, October 1997.

---

which brought together representatives from its local law enforcement, judicial, social services, educational, religious, and medical fields to create a comprehensive program to protect its youngest citizens while encouraging positive, healthful behavior. Other communities, both urban and rural, could adapt these strategies to fit their needs and available resources.

Consistent Enforcement Practices

While community acceptance remains paramount, a juvenile curfew can succeed only if authorities enforce it in a consistent, fair, and uniform manner. To this end, law enforcement agencies should establish curfew enforcement policies that set forth required procedures, including guidelines for confronting potential violators, enforcement options, and reporting and follow-up requirements. Agencies should advise community members of these procedures to ensure their support and compliance. For example, Charlottesville police officers met with parents and guardians of juveniles and explained the procedures that they would follow. The vast majority of parents and guardians told the officers that they fully supported the curfew, and many of them, particularly single mothers of teenagers, said that the curfew would help them restrict their children's activities.

Officers who deal with curfew violators also need to comprehend the various reasons that youngsters may have for committing such acts. For example, Charlottesville officers found that some juveniles had not realized they were out past the curfew, others had run away from home and needed social or child protective services, while still others had engaged in repeated curfew violations for criminal purposes. Therefore, the department established enforcement guidelines and procedures for its officers to follow that included a variety of options—such as telling the violator to proceed directly home, transporting the juvenile home, or arresting and detaining the youngster. Agencies should encourage their officers to use discretion when determining their courses of action and always consider the safety of the violators, as well as the community, when determining which enforcement option to choose.

Accurate Record Keeping

Accurate record keeping stands as an important element of successfully implementing curfews. A complete record should include the number of juveniles contacted as a result of the curfew and the number detained, released, and summoned. Officers should note when and where they found violators; their age, sex, and race; the reason for the violation; and whether the parents or guardians knew the whereabouts of the juveniles. Most important, officers always should document cases where domestic problems or abuse triggered the curfew violation. Charlottesville police officers found this especially true in cases where they may have never learned of such problems, and the youngsters involved may have never received the resultant social services.

The department also found that a follow-up visit, a letter, or even a telephone call by officers assigned to youth activities often prevented future violations. Whichever course officers take, they should document these actions, as well. Likewise, in cases that require the intervention of social or child protection services, officers should record this information and maintain communication with the service provider.

Results

Many communities credit curfews with reducing juvenile crime and violence. Many law enforcement agencies appreciate the tools that curfews give them to keep youths off the streets and away from potential dangers. Many parents and guardians say that they can place boundaries on their children's activities more easily when other young people in the neighborhood must comply with a communitywide curfew. Even though these successful experiences with juvenile curfews exist, critics often oppose such efforts on both practical and legal grounds. However, research has shown that communities can reduce juvenile delinquency and victimization when community members work together to create and implement comprehensive curfew programs.

Since the inception of its curfew, the city of Charlottesville has seen a dramatic decrease in the number of juveniles on the streets late at night or in the early morning hours. While the community experienced relatively little juvenile crime before implementing the curfew, even less has occurred after it began. Most parents and guardians have applauded the police department's efforts of having its school resource officers explain to young people the potential dangers that exist during these time periods. Also, school administrators have noticed an improvement in attendance. Implementing the curfew has gone smoothly, and the results have exceeded the department's expectations of safeguarding the community's children and encouraging them and their families to pursue healthy, constructive lives.

Protecting Children

For over a century, communities in the United States have imposed juvenile curfews to help maintain order and reduce crime committed by youths. Recently, many communities have expanded this basic method of curtailing the activities of young people to include comprehensive, community-based curfew programs, which include strategies to protect children from elements that place them at risk for becoming involved in drugs, gangs, and other dangerous or illegal activities.

To protect its children from such harmful and unhealthy influences, the city of Charlottesville, Virginia, developed and implemented a community-based juvenile curfew program. The community felt that a preventive approach to its young people's wandering the streets late at night or in the early morning hours would prove beneficial in reducing the victimization of these youths. Concern for the safety of its youngsters rather than an increase in juvenile crime propelled the community to implement a curfew program. The success of this effort has shown how community members can work together to find effective ways of not only reducing juvenile crime and violence but, more important, preventing such occurrences in the first place.

> *"If a young person is prepared to commit a burglary, robbery, battery, or murder, he or she is unlikely to be deterred by the prospect of a curfew citation."*

Curfew Laws Do Not Reduce Teenage Crime and Violence

Jordan C. Budd

Jordan C. Budd, managing attorney of the American Civil Liberties Union (ACLU) foundation in San Diego, California, argues in the following viewpoint that curfews fail to reduce the incidence of teenage crime and violence. He contends that most acts of youth crime occur between 3 P.M. and 6 P.M., when most curfew laws are not in effect. In addition, Budd maintains that curfew laws violate juveniles' constitutional rights.

As you read, consider the following questions:
1. According to the author, why will curfew laws most likely affect law-abiding teenagers rather than criminal teenagers?
2. What fundamental rights do curfew laws violate, according to Budd?
3. As cited by the author, what is the difference between "strict scrutiny" and "intermediate scrutiny"?

Jordan C. Budd, "Juvenile Curfews: The Rights of Minors vs. the Rhetoric of Public Safety," *Human Rights*, vol. 26, Fall 1999, pp. 22–24. Copyright © 1999 by American Bar Association. Reproduced by permission.

After an absence of several decades, juvenile curfews have reappeared in communities across the United States. Researchers estimate that nearly 75 percent of major American cities now enforce some form of a nocturnal curfew. As curfews become more widespread, the debate over their efficacy and constitutionality has intensified. That debate frames a number of fundamental questions regarding the relationship between individual liberty and community safety, and the degree to which we are willing to infringe the rights of a discrete and vulnerable group to advance our collective sense of security.

Questionable Efficacy

The premise of juvenile curfews—that serious criminal activity among youths will decline if they are barred from leaving their homes—has a simple and intuitive appeal. Yet, the most severe sanction found anywhere for a curfew violation is a criminal misdemeanor charge—hardly a deterrent for youths willing to risk the far more onerous penalties that attach to the type of crimes curfews seek to prevent. Quite simply, if a young person is prepared to commit a burglary, robbery, battery, or murder, he or she is unlikely to be deterred by the prospect of a curfew citation. Conversely, law-abiding youths will likely modify their conduct to conform to the law, even if it requires that they forego socially productive activities. By their design, curfews will have the greatest impact on the conduct of those youth with whom we are least concerned.

No empirical research has yet demonstrated that curfews have any appreciable effect on rates of juvenile crime. After reviewing available literature and data concerning the efficacy of juvenile curfews in major American cities, two scholars concluded in 1995 that "there is so little existing research on the effects of curfews that policymakers have next to nothing to guide them concerning the benefits and costs of a curfew." What limited evidence does exist provides little support for curfew enforcement. A 1998 study of juvenile curfews in California, which compared the rate of juvenile crime in jurisdictions with curfews against the rate of crime elsewhere, concluded that "curfew enforcement generally had no discernible effect on youth crime."

In the absence of empirical data, cities often cite a general decline in crime rates over the period during which a curfew is enforced as proof that it works, without any attempt to control for demographic, economic, or social influences. Indeed, in correlating declining crime with curfew enforcement, curfew proponents often fail to make the most basic distinction between crime occurring during curfew hours and crime occurring at other times of the day. The statistical arguments advanced by the City of San Diego in support of its juvenile curfew are illustrative. Citing an overall drop in arrests for juvenile crime during the first year of San Diego's curfew enforcement program (1995), the city declared that its curfew was a success. The data actually demonstrated that the violent crime rate during curfew hours remained essentially unchanged (233 arrests in 1994; 222 arrests in 1995), while the crime rate during noncurfew hours plummeted (1,501 arrests in 1994; 1,224 arrests in 1995). San Diego thus credited its juvenile curfew with a decline in crime that occurred almost entirely during the period when the curfew was not in effect.

Moreover, less than 15 percent of all arrests for violent juvenile crime in San Diego occur during curfew hours, consistent with national data indicating that juvenile crime peaks at 3:00 P.M. and again at 6:00 P.M.—well before curfews take effect. Therefore, even if curfews were effective, they would reach only a small percentage of the violent juvenile crime in the community. Perhaps most significantly, juvenile crime in its entirety accounts for less than 10 percent of all violent crime committed in the United States. Nocturnal juvenile curfews thus target a relatively small portion of the criminal landscape—likely less than 2 percent of all violent crime.

Demonizing Our Youth

The lack of data establishing the efficacy of curfews has not diminished their political appeal. Juvenile curfews speak to our collective fear of the dangers lurking in the night, and target an easily caricatured culprit class. A 1994 survey of 300 adult residents in Cincinnati revealed that 92 percent supported the city's juvenile curfew, 72 percent agreed that the curfew made them feel safer, and 87 percent believed that the curfew helped control delinquency. The image of dissolute youth roaming the streets in search of victims is now a fixture of our political rhetoric, and curfews offer a satisfying and uncomplicated solution.

Demonizing our youth—the vast majority of whom obey the law, work hard, and make positive contributions to their families and communities—is not without cost, as the young people who brought the legal challenge to San Diego's juvenile curfew demonstrate. One 17-year-old plaintiff volunteered each week to work in the kitchen of a downtown homeless shelter. Because meals were served after dark, when the homeless population returned from the streets, she regularly returned home after 10:00 P.M. and, as a result, was forced to quit when the curfew was enacted. Another plaintiff was an aspiring actor who traveled by train to Los Angeles to audition for parts in theatrical productions. Because he typically returned to San Diego from auditions after 10:00 P.M., he was in violation of the law. Yet another plaintiff was required to cancel the study sessions she held in the evenings with other students at a local coffeehouse to prepare for Advanced Placement exams. Each of these youths acted with the permission and encouragement of their parents but nonetheless invited a criminal citation for their activities—as did their complicit parents.

Constitutional Implications

Even if the efficacy of curfews were established, and their popularity justified as something more than political scapegoating, the most troubling questions regarding curfew enforcement would remain. If we empower law enforcement to empty the streets of all persons—adults as well as juveniles—between 10:00 P.M. and sunrise, perhaps crime will occur less frequently, at least during that time period. The objection, of course, is that such an enforcement tactic vests police with inordinate, unchecked power, which offends our most basic sense of liberty and autonomy, and is simply too high a price to pay in a free society for an incremental decrease in crime rates.

Opponents of juvenile curfews pose the same objection.

In implementing curfews, cities entrust their police with vast discretion to enforce a law that specifies nothing more than youthful appearance as probable cause for detention. Anyone who looks remotely close to 18 years of age is fair game for an investigatory stop and interrogation. Because police lack the resources and often the motivation to stop every person on the street who might pass for a teenager, officers necessarily will select curfew suspects on the basis of additional considerations, which may include race, class, and other biases—giving them carte blanche to engage in arbitrary and discriminatory enforcement practices.

Juvenile curfews are constitutionally suspect in a more fundamental respect as well. Curfews aim to prevent criminal activity before it occurs through the preemptive detention of all potential offenders, along with every other law-abiding young person in the jurisdiction. Such a blunt and overreaching crime-fighting technique would plainly be unenforceable against adults. . . . The question then becomes whether the rights of minors are sufficiently different to warrant such sweeping and arbitrary regulation. The U.S. Supreme Court has not ruled on the issue, and the lower courts have reached widely divergent conclusions.

Fundamental Rights

Because juvenile curfews burden a variety of fundamental rights (e.g., the right to free speech and association, the right to free movement, the right to travel, and the right to free exercise of religion), the analysis of curfew laws is a complex exercise involving the application of a number of different constitutional standards and doctrines. At the center of the judicial debate, however, is one common issue: whether the constitutional rights of minors are sufficiently "fundamental" to warrant strict scrutiny review for purposes of equal protection analysis. Strict scrutiny requires that any measure infringing the fundamental rights of an adult class be narrowly tailored to promote a compelling governmental interest. Some courts have held that this protective standard applies to the rights of minors as well—and, not surprisingly, have struck down curfews as a result.

In considering a challenge to San Diego's juvenile curfew,

the Ninth Circuit ruled that "rights are no less 'fundamental' for minors than adults" and thus the curfew was subject to strict scrutiny review. While acknowledging that "minors' rights are not coextensive with the rights of adults because the state has a greater range of [compelling] interests that justify the infringement of minors' rights"—thus permitting driving restrictions, compulsory education laws, prohibitions against alcohol consumption, and other targeted limitations on the autonomy of youths—the court concluded that San Diego's curfew was not narrowly tailored to advance the city's interests. Other courts have similarly employed strict scrutiny analysis to strike down curfews as overbroad restrictions on the fundamental rights of young people.

Curfews Hurt Law-Abiding Teens

In Washington, D.C., a law keeps people under 17 at home from 11 P.M. to 6 A.M. on weeknights and from midnight to 6 A.M. on weekends. . . . A 17-year-old member of two musical bands said his town's curfew kept him from participating in evening performances. A 15-year-old competitive swimmer noted that he has to leave his house at 4:45 A.M.—while the curfew is in effect—to practice with his team. A 16-year-old complained about being unable to participate in informal study groups after curfew hours. A 14-year-old was upset that he couldn't engage, legally, in a number of social activities, such as stopping to get something to eat after a debate tournament, going to the opera with his 18-year-old sister, and watching late-night movies with his friends.

Margaret Davidson, *Reason*, November 1999.

Given the inherent breadth of any curfew law, which necessarily places every law-abiding youth under some form of home detention so that a relatively small number of serious juvenile offenders might remain inside as well, it is difficult to envision how such an enactment could be deemed "narrowly tailored" to advance the government's interest in averting youth crime. Strict scrutiny review, therefore, presents a serious hurdle for curfew proponents. The Fourth and D.C. Circuits addressed this difficulty by adopting an entirely different analytic approach. Rejecting the proposition that the rights of juveniles are sufficiently fundamental to warrant strict scrutiny review, these courts have ruled that juveniles are entitled only to intermediate scrutiny of laws that infringe their "qualified rights." Intermediate scrutiny requires only that a law be substantially related to an important government interest. In both cases, the challenged curfews were upheld under the more lenient standard as "substantially" related to the government's interest in controlling juvenile crime.

The application of intermediate scrutiny rescues juvenile curfews from their inherent constitutional infirmities by relieving government of the obligation to narrowly craft laws that impinge on the fundamental rights of minors. By formally excluding minors from the full reach of the Constitution, the application of intermediate scrutiny permits the enactment of sweeping regulations that punish innocent and law-abiding youth for the sins of a few among them. As Judge David S. Tatel of the Fourth Circuit wrote in dissent,

> [the majority's analysis] relegates kids to second-class citizenship. . . . As long as the majority's standard is the law, a city council can pass a juvenile curfew as a routine measure because the justification is so easy to articulate. This should not stand under the Constitution. Children make up a quarter of our population, and their rights must not be ignored. A city council cannot order such a large segment of the community to stay at home for thirty-three hours of every week unless its curfew satisfies strict scrutiny.

If embraced in other contexts, this precedent could alter substantially the nature of juveniles' constitutional protections and significantly expand the government's ability to infringe and potentially abuse the interests of young people. To do such damages to the fundamental rights of youths in the service of a public policy of such poor design and doubtful efficacy is especially ironic.

False Sense of Safety

There is little evidence that curfews have any appreciable effect on juvenile crime rates. They likely have the greatest impact on the activities of those youths who are least likely to commit crimes, and bar them from engaging in a variety of socially productive activities. By their design, curfews vest law enforcement with immense and unreviewable power to engage in arbitrary enforcement practices, and punish all law-abiding youth for the transgressions of a few among them.

To secure constitutional sanction for this sweeping law enforcement practice, courts have excluded minors from the full reach of the Constitution and have held that the infringement of their rights is subject to less demanding scrutiny than the impairment of the rights of adults. We pay a very high price for the illusory sense of safety that juvenile curfews provide.

5

> "*School administrators can, and should,
> have no tolerance for threats of violence
> and should react swiftly to them.*"

Zero Tolerance Laws Reduce Teen Crime and Violence

Vito A. Gagliardi Jr.

In the following viewpoint, Vito A. Gagliardi Jr. argues that zero tolerance laws can help teachers and school administrators fight teenage crime and violence. Citing from New Jersey's zero tolerance statute, Gagliardi contends that under this policy any student who is caught with a firearm or assaults a member of the school staff will be expelled. Gagliardi maintains that if these policies are observed fairly at all schools, they may prevent future acts of violence on campus. Gagliardi, an attorney in New Jersey, represents school boards.

As you read, consider the following questions:

1. What did the Improving America's Schools Act of 1994 mandate, according to the author?
2. According to Gagliardi, how has the notion of zero tolerance expanded since the laws were enacted?
3. As stated by the author, why does "one size not fit all"?

Vito A. Gagliardi Jr., "In Defense of Zero Tolerance," *New Jersey Law Journal*, vol. 164, May 21, 2001, p. 27. Copyright © 2001 by ALM Properties, Inc. Reproduced by permission.

New Jersey schools' "zero tolerance" for violence and threats of violence is the subject of much discussion in the classroom and the courtroom. Unfortunately, such discussions include criticism based on a misunderstanding, and occasional misapplication, of the laws as "one-size-punishment-fits-all" solutions to complex problems.

We have all read of the rigid application of the laws, for example, to expel first graders because they pretended their fingers were weapons in a playground game of cops and robbers. In reality, however, these laws are flexible enough to consider mitigating factors in students' behaviors when warranted.

The Rise of Zero Tolerance

The statutes known as the "zero tolerance" laws were passed in 1995 as a part of New Jersey's efforts to comply with then-new federal law, the Improving America's Schools Act (IASA) of 1994. The IASA mandated that states require local education agencies to "expel" from school for a period of not less than one year any pupil who brought a weapon to school.

The federal law did not define the term "expulsion," and the New Jersey Legislature determined that "removal" of pupils for violations would comply with the intent of the federal law.

In addition to revising the existing statute prohibiting the assault of staff members, the Legislature passed two additional statutes in 1995, known as the "Zero Tolerance for Guns Act," which read as follows:

> Any pupil who is convicted or adjudicated delinquent for possession of a firearm or a crime while armed with a firearm or found knowingly in possession of a firearm on any school property, on a school bus, or at a school-sponsored function shall be immediately removed from the school's regular education program pending a hearing before the local board of education to remove the pupil from the regular education program for a period of not less than one calendar year subject to modification on a case-by-case basis by the chief school administrator.

> Any pupil who commits an assault upon a teacher, administrator, board member, other employee of the school board or another student, with a weapon, on any school property, on a school bus, or at a school-sponsored function shall be im-

mediately removed from the school's regular education program pending a hearing before the local board of education.

Both laws took effect for the 1995–1996 school year.

Any pupils accused of violating these statutes are entitled to a hearing before the board of education no later than 30 calendar days after his or her removal from the regular educational program. According to the statutes, any pupil removed from the educational program "shall be placed in an alternative educational program. If placement in an alternative educational program is not available, the pupil shall be provided home instructions or other suitable facilities and programs until placement is available."

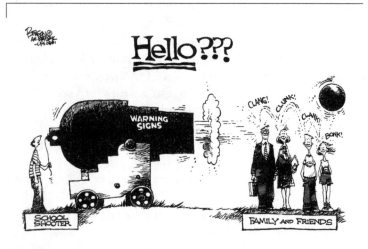

Benson. © 2001 by United Feature Syndicate. Reprinted with permission.

The principal is responsible for the immediate removal of the pupil pending the hearing, and the principal has the option to suspend the student for up to 10 school days pending the hearing and/or placement through other arrangements. (These procedures apply specifically to nonclassified students; students classified as eligible for special education are entitled to a comprehensive range of additional procedures that are not addressed here.)

Significantly, the chief school administrator, in most districts the superintendent of schools, can modify any decision to remove a pupil on a case-by-case basis. Further, the statutes specifically reserve the right of the chief school administrator to determine whether the pupil is prepared to return to the regular educational program or whether the pupil must remain in the alternative educational program or other educational placement.

The Expanding Notion of Zero Tolerance

In the . . . years since these laws were enacted, the notion of zero tolerance has expanded in the minds of many individuals, although not in the laws themselves. Now, threats made through e-mails, notes and anonymous scrollings on bathroom walls are all met with zero tolerance. These days, school districts cannot take lightly simple written or verbal threats, which years ago would have been ignored.

More specifically, since these laws were originally passed, students have used weapons to kill and injure classmates and staff members throughout the United States. Consider the infamy visited on the following towns from 1995 to 2001: Pearl, Mississippi; West Paducah, Kentucky; Jonesboro, Arkansas; Fayetteville, Tennessee; Springfield, Oregon; Littleton, Colorado; Conyers, Georgia; Demming, New Mexico; and Fort Gibson, Oklahoma. In most of these instances, just as in the case of the tragedy at Santana High School in California in March 2001, there were warning signs that the violent youngsters were considering doing something dramatic.

We must allow school administrators the flexibility to act before the weapons appear on the scene and lead to the carnage they have so frequently caused. Thus, school administrators can, and should, have no tolerance for threats of violence and should react swiftly to them.

However, this does not mean that they can, or should, overreact. Every incident must be investigated and every student should be given all the due process required by law. Occasionally, school administrators are best served by having the police investigate a situation. And, be they threats investigated by school administrators or police, the punishment should fit the crime.

In my experience in representing numerous, diverse school districts during the past 10 years, I have learned that even the silliest threats must be taken seriously.

Occasionally a student who is making "jokes" about committing a violent act is reported to the police, who eventually find that the youngster was stockpiling weapons, had access to dad's gun or was making plans to carry out this threat, which would have been discovered much too late if school administrators had not acted on the threat alone.

One Size Does Not Fit All

Recently, the American Bar Association (ABA) issued a report calling for the repeal of zero tolerance laws: "Zero tolerance has become a one-size-fits-all solution to all problems that schools confront. It has redefined students as criminals with unfortunate consequences."

The ABA would be right, if its underlying assumption were true. One size does not fit all. Indeed, school officials have always had the authority to discipline, and even expel, students whose conduct constitutes a continuing danger to the physical well-being of others. The notion of zero tolerance for weapons and serious threats has changed only the idea of what should be punished and how punishment should be meted out.

However, one thing has not changed. Professional educators are in the best position to determine what needs to be done to keep their schools safe. The law gives them the flexibility to respond to each case on an individualized basis.

Of course, there will be times when even the most well-intentioned school administrator acts too hastily. That does not mean that these laws should be eliminated when we need them most. What it means is that our courts will have to remedy the occasional overreaction, which is one of the reasons they are there in the first place.

"I've read dozens of news stories about outrageously stupid acts of school discipline."

Zero Tolerance Laws Are Unfair

James Taranto

Zero tolerance laws vary across schools, but they generally suspend, expel, or jail students who are caught with a potential weapon on campus. James Taranto, editor of *OpinionJournal.com*, an online resource for *Wall Street Journal* editorials, argues in the following viewpoint that zero tolerance laws unfairly punish teenagers for trivial offenses, such as drawing pictures of weapons or pointing toy guns at classmates. Taranto contends that zero tolerance laws have caused more hysteria at schools than the presence of real knives and guns.

As you read, consider the following questions:
1. According to the author, why was Kara Williams suspended?
2. What was the child who pointed a toy gun at his classmate charged with, as stated by Taranto?
3. What are the odds of being killed at school, as reported by the author?

Quick: Name an issue that unites the liberal American Civil Liberties Union (ACLU) and the conservative Rutherford Institute. The answer is "zero tolerance," the lunatic policy under which schools across America are suspending, expelling and even jailing kids for the most trivial of offenses, all in the name of preventing another [school shooting like] Columbine [where fifteen people were killed in 1999].

On May 4, 2001, the ACLU won a temporary restraining order on behalf of Kara Williams, a 16-year-old freshman at Rio Rancho High School, near Albuquerque, New Mexico. Ms. Williams had the misfortune of being out of class at a time when two other girls were suspected of smoking marijuana in the girls' room. She was summoned to the principal's office, where a security guard searched her bag. She had no pot, but the guard did find a key chain, attached to which was a tiny penknife, complete with tweezers, toothpick and a one-inch blade.

Under the school's zero tolerance weapons policy, Ms. Williams was suspended for the remainder of the school year—some 45 days. Five weeks later, federal judge Bruce Black ordered the school to readmit Kara pending the outcome of the case; last week the school board effectively reduced her sentence to time served.

But the allegation of "carrying a deadly weapon" will remain on her record, unless Judge Black rules otherwise. Deadly? Ms. Williams's stepfather told KOAT-TV that he brought a similar penknife to the federal courthouse, where a security officer "looked at it and didn't think nothing of it. Went through the metal detector, gave it back to me and said, 'Go on.'"

The Case of the Sketch

The Rutherford Institute, meanwhile, has filed a federal lawsuit on behalf of nine-year-old Raleigh "Trey" Walker III, suspended for drawing weapons. That's *drawing*—as in illustrating, sketching, depicting. In March 2001, Trey, a third-grader at Lenwil Elementary School in West Monroe, Louisiana, drew a picture of a soldier holding a knife—a tribute, his father said, to a relative in the Army. Principal

Edward Davis put Trey on "in-school suspension" for a day, saying he found the picture upsetting. "We can't tolerate anything that has to do with guns or knives," Mr. Davis told the *Monroe News-Star*.

Zero Tolerance Laws Defy Commonsense

Every day throughout the United States, children are being shut out of the education system through the application of Zero Tolerance Policies. These policies require that children in kindergarten through 12th grade receive harsh punishments, often for minor infractions that pose no threat to safety, and yet cause them and their families severe hardship. A strong body of compelling research indicates that these "get-tough" disciplinary measures often fail to meet sound educational principles and, in many cases, their application simply defies commonsense. More alarming than the punishment meted out in schools is the tracking of children into the juvenile justice system for minor misconduct in school. Often African-American, Latino, and disabled children bear the brunt of the consequences of these policies. Policymakers, educators, and parents should be very concerned with the long-term implications of denying educational opportunities to millions of children, particularly when the effectiveness of these policies in ensuring school safety is highly suspect.

The Advancement Project and the Civil Rights Project, "Opportunities Suspended: The Devastating Consequences of Zero Tolerance and School Discipline Policies," June 2000.

Willie Isby, director of child welfare and attendance for the Ouachita Parish school system, added that "the punishment is not that bad in this case, in light of the fact that we have been having all these killings in schools." Mr. Isby also vowed to suppress "copycat drawings." Meanwhile Trey's father, Raleigh Walker II, told the *News-Star*, "I had to explain to him that owning guns and being in the Army is not bad."

Stupid Acts of School Discipline

Since March, 2001, when I began following zero-tolerance . . . , I've read dozens of news stories about outrageously stupid acts of school discipline. Here's a sampling:

• In May 2001, an 11-year-old fifth-grader in Oldsmar, Florida, was hauled out of class in handcuffs for drawing pictures of weapons. "The children were in no danger at all," Oldsmar Elementary Principal David Schmitt acknowledged in an interview with the *St. Petersburg Times*. "It involved no real weapons." But school-district spokesman Ron Stone told the *Times* that handcuffing is "normal procedure in a situation like this."

• A 16-year-old girl was suspended for 10 days from Pau-Wa-Lu Middle School in Gardnerville, Nevada, for compiling a list of classmates who "frustrated" her. "We don't want a school shooting in our county, and we would rather err on the side of student safety," principal Robbin Pedrett told the Associated Press—even though the girl had no access to weapons.

• In Stuart, Florida, a nine-year-old second-grader was arrested and charged with aggravated assault—a felony—after he allegedly pointed a toy gun at a classmate at J.D. Parker Elementary School. Earlier, two eight-year-olds at the Augusta Street School in Irvington, New Jersey, were charged with "making terrorist threats" after playing cops and robbers with "paper guns." (Prosecutors later dropped the charges.) And in Jonesboro, Arkansas, eight-year-old Christopher Kissinger was suspended from South Elementary School for three days for pointing a boneless, breaded chicken finger at a teacher and saying, "Pow, pow, pow."

Criminalizing Ordinary Behavior

What accounts for this madness? Why are schools so wildly overreacting to, or even criminalizing, ordinary juvenile behavior? The specter of Columbine and other heavily publicized school shootings obviously haunts school officials everywhere. But zero tolerance long predates that massacre. The Education Department reported that in the 1996–97 school year—two years before Columbine—94% of schools nationwide already had zero tolerance policies for firearms.

The reactions we've seen lately—reminiscent of the Secret Service investigating every wisecrack or offhand remark about assassinating the president—are vastly disproportionate to the actual risk. The Secret Service has reason to be hypervigilant. Of the 42 men who have served as president, four were assassinated and another six survived at least one assassination attempt. If you're president, then, the odds of your being an assassination target are 23.8%, or nearly one in four. The likelihood of being killed in school is more like one in two million, or 0.00005%.

The Associated Press reported in May 2001 that the Columbine Review Commission, set up by Governor Bill Owens in the wake of the 1999 massacre, is recommending that every Colorado high school set up a team to evaluate verbal and written threats. Perhaps these teams will approach the task with sensitivity and common sense. But if the stories we've seen from around the country are any indication, America's schoolchildren have more to fear from mass hysteria in the name of zero tolerance than from any lack of vigilance on the part of school officials.

Periodical Bibliography

The following articles have been selected to supplement the diverse views presented in this chapter.

Vikas Bajaj   "Locking Up Juveniles for Life Not the Answer," *State News*, April 1, 1998.

Michael Bochenek   "United States Must Do Part to Stop Executions of Juvenile Criminals," *Atlanta Journal-Constitution*, August 22, 2000.

Jeffrey Butts and   "One-Size-Fits-All Justice Simply Isn't Fair,
Adele Harrell   Should the Punishment Fit the Crime or the Offender? Trying Kids as Adults Is a 'Get-Tough' Overreaction," *Christian Science Monitor*, December 1, 1998.

Delbert S. Elliott   "Put Greater Focus on Prevention," *USA Today*, June 21, 1999.

T. Markus Funk   "Adult Treatment Fits 'Predators,'" *San Francisco Chronicle*, July 7, 1997.

Dave Grossman   "Teaching Kids to Kill," *Phi Kappa Phi Journal*, Fall 2000.

Darlene Kennedy   "Let's Hold Juveniles Responsible for Their Crimes," *National Policy Analysis*, August 1997.

Charles Levandosky   "House Passes Its Own Abominable Crime Bill," *Liberal Opinion Week*, August 9, 1999.

Robyn Nordell   "Curfew Laws Violate Our Constitutional Rights," *Orange County Register*, January 7, 1998.

Geneva Overholser   "Tough on Crime, Care for Kids," *Washington Post*, January 18, 2000.

William S. Pollack   "The Columbine Syndrome," *National Forum*, Fall 2000.

Amy Tay   "Curfew Today, Bedtime Tomorrow?" *Los Angeles Times*, February 8, 1998.

Walter E. Williams   "Making a Case for Corporal Punishment," *Insight*, September 13, 1999.

Jason Ziedenberg and   "The Risks Juveniles Face," *Corrections Today*,
Vincent Schiraldi   August 1998.

CHAPTER 4

How Can Teen Substance Abuse Be Reduced?

Chapter Preface

Almost all teenagers have some experience with alcohol, drugs, and tobacco. Most teens will experiment with substances and stop. However, some will continue to use regularly and display different degrees of emotional, physical, and social problems, such as difficulty in school or family tension. Some teens will become dependent on a substance and be destructive to themselves or others. Some will die or cause others to die in drug- or alcohol-related incidents. However, there is no certain way to predict which teens will develop serious problems as a result of experimenting with drugs, alcohol, or tobacco. Therefore, all teen substance use must be regarded as potentially dangerous.

According to a 2002 survey by the National Center on Addiction and Substance Abuse at Columbia University, most teens who use alcohol, cigarettes, and marijuana do so before they are fifteen years old. By the age of fifteen, the study found, 95 percent of teenagers have had their first cigarette, 93 percent have had their first alcoholic drink, and 86 percent have tried marijuana. The Centers for Disease Control and Prevention (CDC) reports that about three thousand adolescents start smoking every day, and roughly one thousand of them will become addicted to nicotine. Another study found that almost all high school seniors have used alcohol, and two-thirds reported that they had used it in the last month. A survey of seventeen thousand high school seniors found that nearly 33 percent had taken at least one illicit drug during the preceding year.

Substance abuse can have enormous consequences on a teenager's physical, emotional, and psychological health. Adolescent smoking, for example, puts teens at risk for lung cancer, chronic bronchitis, emphysema, heart attacks, high blood pressure, strokes, and arteriosclerosis later in life. In addition, teen smokers suffer decreased lung capacity, causing shortness of breath and reduced stamina. Alcohol and drug abuse also threaten teens' well-being, primarily because being intoxicated hinders good judgment. "That puts you at risk for making poor life decisions," contends Alan Leshner, director of the National Institute on Drug Abuse.

For example, teens under the influence of drugs or alcohol are more likely to engage in fights, destruction of property, date rapes, car accidents, and unprotected sex—which can lead to unwanted pregnancies and sexually transmitted diseases—than teens who are not under the influence.

Experts agree that it is impossible to predict which teens will develop serious problems as a result of substance use, but several factors put some teenagers at greater risk of abusing drugs or alcohol. For instance, teens with family members who smoke cigarettes, drink alcohol, or use drugs are more likely to become addicted to a substance than teens whose family members do not use these substances. In addition, experts associate teen substance abuse with inadequate parental supervision and poor interaction between parents and teens. When parents are not involved in their adolescent's life, addiction specialists maintain, the teen has more freedom to engage in risky behaviors. Family conflict also contributes to teen substance abuse; experts contend that some teenagers seek to deaden the pain of physical, emotional, or sexual abuse in the home with drugs or alcohol. Other factors that contribute to teen substance abuse include rebellion, poor impulse control, and peer pressure, among others.

Finding solutions to the problem of teen substance abuse is a pressing social issue. Authors in the following chapter debate ways to help teenagers avoid the lure of alcohol, drugs, and tobacco.

"[A consequence of the minimum drinking age] is that a lot fewer teenagers now end their lives in alcohol-related traffic accidents."

Age Restrictions on Alcohol Reduce Teen Drinking

Steve Chapman

In the following viewpoint, Steve Chapman contends that age restrictions on alcohol consumption have significantly reduced the number of drunk-driving deaths among teens. If the drinking age were lowered to eighteen, he argues, eighteen-year-olds would be free to buy alcohol for much younger teens. Chapman maintains that age restrictions on alcohol are not a perfect solution to the problem of teen drinking, but they cause less damage to society than lowering the drinking age would. Chapman is a columnist and editorial writer for the *Chicago Tribune*.

As you read, consider the following questions:
1. As reported by Chapman, what did the alcohol-related 1984 federal law mandate?
2. Which sect of society opposes lowering the drinking age, according to the author?
3. As stated by the author, how do lax state liquor laws affect other states?

Steve Chapman, "Keep the Drinking Age at 21," *Weekly Standard*, July 30, 2001, pp. 15–16. Copyright © 2001 by *Weekly Standard*. Reproduced by permission.

Between [the 1999 shootings at] Columbine [high school in Colorado], rapper Eminem, and MTV, today's teenagers often come across to their elders as indecent, self-destructive, and dangerous. But Baby Boomers shouldn't be too quick to judge. In one respect, modern adolescents behave far more responsibly than their parents did at the same age. High school students today are far less likely to drink or to drink and drive.

Help from the Folks

This is partly because of changing attitudes among kids. But they've also gotten some crucial help from adults—particularly a 1984 law effectively forcing every state to bar alcohol sales to anyone under the age of 21. One consequence is that a lot fewer teenagers now end their lives in alcohol-related traffic accidents. Since 1982, the number of youngsters killed in crashes involving a drunken teenage driver has plunged by 63 percent. The National Highway Traffic Safety Administration [NHTSA] estimates that higher drinking ages have saved more than 19,000 lives since 1975—including 901 in 1999. "Drinking and driving," reports NHTSA, "is no longer the leading cause of death for teenagers."

But a lot of people count that as a piddling achievement. Since President George W. Bush's 19-year-old daughters were cited for trying to buy alcohol at an Austin establishment, a chorus has gone up in favor of lowering the drinking age. And a lot of the voices have come from the right. Conservative columnist Kathleen Parker, writing in *USA Today*, noted that Jenna Bush can legally vote, go to war, get an abortion, get married, and be prosecuted as an adult—"yet we insist that when it comes to alcohol, she conduct herself as a child." An op-ed piece in the *Wall Street Journal* assailed the current law as "irrational" and "morally confused." Even the *Economist* magazine weighed in, attributing the 21-year age floor to two malign currents in American life: "petty puritanism and a pathological obsession with safety."

Surprising Support

One group has conspicuously dissented from the emerging new consensus: the people who would be most affected by the change. A recent poll by the survey organization Institute for Creative Research (ICR) found that 84 percent of teenagers support keeping or raising the current drinking age. "In a given year, the majority of high school seniors drink, but only a small proportion are drinking heavily," Boston University School of Public Health scholar Ralph Hingson told the Associated Press. "On balance, they are supportive of legislation that will reduce the risks to themselves."

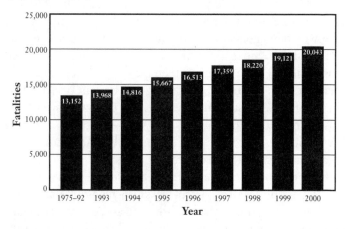

Cumulative Estimated Number of Lives Saved by Minimum Drinking Age Laws, 1975–2000

National Highway Traffic Safety Administration, 2002.

So why would anyone want to increase the risks to them? Simple consistency, we are told, demands a change. If 18-year-olds are adults for purposes of voting, enlisting in the military, signing contracts, and most everything else, the argument goes, they should certainly be free to go into a restaurant and order a margarita. The Bush daughters were only doing what most young people do sooner or later—trying to circumvent a law that denies them a simple and often harmless adult pleasure. Treat 18-year-olds like grown-ups, and they'll act more like grown-ups.

But this is one of those instances that bring to mind the supremely conservative observation of Justice Oliver Wendell Holmes Jr.: "A page of history is worth a volume of logic." We raised the drinking age in the 1980s not because we were eager to turn college campuses into monasteries, but because we could no longer stomach the costs incurred when many states lowered their drinking age in the 1970s. Thanks to that change, alcohol-related highway deaths rose, helping to fuel the rise of Mothers Against Drunk Driving and a broad national effort to reduce the carnage. If we abandon the 21-year drinking age, we can expect to forfeit a lot of lives, both young and old.

Practical Considerations

A uniform age of consent holds a superficial appeal, but practical considerations ought to weigh heavily in our calculations. There are good reasons to treat 18-year-olds differently for different purposes. Some responsibilities they are ready for. Others they may not be. Experience suggests that teenagers may be trusted to drive a car. But drinking and driving are another story entirely. A one-size-fits-all policy pretends that the world is a neater place than the complicated reality we know.

Another argument against foolish consistency is that the drinking age is a uniquely porous barrier. Lowering the voting age to 18 didn't cause a mass outbreak of illegal voting by 15-year-olds. Very few high school students obtain fake IDs so they can take out a mortgage or join the Navy before the law allows. But many, if not most, are fiercely impatient when it comes to alcohol. Setting the drinking age at 21 can be criticized as a highly imperfect way of keeping booze away from college-age kids, who have devised numerous ways to get it. But it does hinder them at least a little. Perhaps more important, the existing law presents even greater obstacles for younger teens. Lower the floor to 18, and millions of high school seniors would suddenly be free to buy all the Budweiser their friends can guzzle. Middle schoolers would soon find alcohol more accessible than it is today. Drinking among adolescents has fallen substantially in the last 20 years. If we want to take it upon ourselves to reverse that trend, reducing the drinking age is a sure way to do it.

Conservatives argue that in any event, this is a matter that ought to be handled through state decisions, not by federal coercion. But federalism, correctly understood, doesn't mean leaving all decisions to the states—only those decisions whose consequences are largely confined within their boundaries. If California chooses to bar construction of power generators or New York levies high taxes, its citizens will pay the price. But we don't let one state foul the air of its neighbors at will, or block goods and services coming from elsewhere. In those sorts of cases, the federal government steps in, as it should.

Like air pollution, lax liquor laws reach insidiously across borders. Back when there was no national uniformity, some states, such as Wisconsin, allowed 18-year-olds to drink, while others, such as neighboring Illinois, didn't. So taverns just north of the interstate border promoted heavily to bring in Illinoisans who were just a short trip away from beer heaven. Many of them accepted the invitation, took full advantage of Wisconsin's hospitality, and then perished trying to drive home in a fog of alcohol. The Wisconsin-Illinois line became known as the "blood border." Let states regain control over the drinking age, and that grim history will repeat itself.

Sterile Attitudes

An economist was once defined as someone who, upon seeing something work fine in practice, wonders if it can work in theory. A similarly sterile attitude afflicts those who want to lower the drinking age. Conservatives should be the last people to elevate blind consistency over prudent accommodations of reality. Keeping the current drinking age is contradictory, less than satisfying, and, in some sense, unfair. But it's far preferable to an approach that is logical, uniform, and wrong.

> "Demonizing alcohol—and thus elevating
> it to the status of forbidden fruit—is
> counterproductive."

Age Restrictions on Alcohol Do Not Reduce Teen Drinking

Andrew Stuttaford

In the following viewpoint, Andrew Stuttaford argues that age restrictions on drinking alcohol are ineffective and counterproductive. He contends that underage drinking laws, by making drinking taboo, make consuming alcohol more attractive to teens, and thus encourage more underage drinking. He maintains that teen alcohol consumption can best be reduced by strengthening the deterrents, not trying to enforce an indefensible drinking law. Stuttaford is a contributor to the *National Review*.

As you read, consider the following questions:
1. What recent efforts has Texas made to reduce the incidence of teenage drinking, as stated by the author?
2. According to Stuttaford, how should parents introduce their teens to responsible drinking?
3. How has the minimum drinking age affected drunk driving rates, as reported by the author?

It was a day of shame for the Bushes, an incident made all the more embarrassing by the family's previous well-publicized difficulties with alcohol. I refer, of course, to the regrettable 1997 decision by then-governor George W. Bush to approve legislation further toughening the penalties for underage drinking. In Texas, the legal drinking age is 21. A typical Texan of 19—let's call her "Jenna"—is judged to be responsible enough to vote, drive, marry, serve in the military, and (this is Texas) be executed, but she is not, apparently, sufficiently mature to decide for herself whether to buy a margarita.[1] The 1997 legislation made things worse: Miller Time could now mean hard time, a possible six months in jail for a third offense.

Remnants of Prohibition

It is a ludicrous and demeaning law, but it has been policed with all the gung-ho enthusiasm that we have come to expect in a land where the prohibitionist impulse has never quite died. In Austin, Texas, there is now a special squad of undercover cops dedicated to fighting the scourge of teenage tippling. In other words, they hang around in bars.

The crusade does not stop there. The Texas Commission on Alcohol and Drug Abuse boasts a campaign called "2young2drink," which features billboards, a hotline (Denounce your friends!), and a program enticingly known as "Shattered Dreams." Other efforts include the Texas Alcoholic Beverage Commission's sting operations (Make your kid a snoop!) and, for those parents 2stupid2think, a helpful series of danger signs compiled by the Texas Safety Network. One early indicator that your child is drinking may be the "smell of alcohol on [his] breath." Who knew?

But it's unfair to single out Texas. The legal drinking age has been raised to 21 in every state, a dreary legacy of Elizabeth Dole's otherwise unremarkable tenure as President Ronald Reagan's transportation secretary. She is not apologizing; her only regret is that the age of barroom consent was not increased to 24. In her jihad against gin, Mrs. Dole

1. In 2001, President George W. Bush's daughter, Jenna Bush, was accused of using a fake I.D. to try to purchase alcohol. The charges were later dropped.

forgot that the guiding principle of the Reagan administration was supposed to be a reduction in the role of the state.

And, as usual, government is not going to do any good. The only circumstances in which the approach taken by the zero-tolerance zealots could have the faintest chance of success would be in a society where alcohol was a rarity. Zero tolerance has been a disastrous failure in the case of young people and illegal drugs; how can it be expected to work with a product that is available in every mall or corner store? Sooner or later, your child will be confronted with that seductive bottle. The only question is how he is going to deal with it.

Not well, if the Dole approach continues to hold sway. Demonizing alcohol—and thus elevating it to the status of forbidden fruit—is counterproductive. Adult disapproval magically transforms that margarita from a simple pleasure into an especially thrilling act of rebellion.

My parents avoided this error. Growing up in more tolerant England, I could always ask them for a drink, and, fairly frequently, I would even be given one. At least partly as a result, I went through adolescence without feeling any need to drink a pint to make a point. My drinks were for the right reasons. The only recollection I have of any real parental anxiety in this area was when, at the age of about 13, I accepted a brandy from a friend of the family (an alleged murderer, as it happens, but that's another story). The worry was not the drink, but the uninsured glass containing it: antique, priceless, and, as our host explained to my trembling mother, quite irreplaceable. In the event, the glass survived me, and I survived the drink.

Parents Are the Best Judges

Parents, not bureaucrats, are the best judges of how and when their offspring should be permitted to drink. Intelligent parents don't let alcohol become a big deal, a mystery or a battleground. They teach its perils, but its pleasures, too. Have a bottle of wine on the table, and let the kids take a gulp; it will not, I promise, turn them into Frenchmen. Treat a drink as a part of growing up, as something to be savored within a family, rather than guzzled down in some rite to mark passage from that family.

Furthermore, too much of the discussion about alcohol in this country reflects prohibitionist fervor rather than scientific fact. We act as if alcohol were a vice, a degenerate habit that can—at best—be tolerated. In reality, it does not need to be apologized for. Alcohol has been a valuable part of Western culture for thousands of years. It can be abused, sure, but it can inspire as well as intoxicate, illuminate as well as irritate. In excess, the demon drink merits its nickname; in moderation, it can be good for you.

Forbidden Fruit

Although the legal purchase age is twenty-one years, a majority of college students under this age consume alcohol—certainly not a surprise to anyone. When they have the opportunity to drink, they do so in an irresponsible manner because drinking by these youth is seen as an enticing "forbidden fruit," a "badge of rebellion against authority" and a symbol of "adulthood." As a nation we have tried prohibition legislation twice in the past for controlling irresponsible drinking problems, during National Prohibition in the 1920s and state prohibition during the 1850s. Because they were unenforceable and because the backlash towards them caused other social problems, these laws were finally repealed.

Prohibition did not work then and prohibition for young people under the age of twenty-one is not working now.

Ruth Engs, *Vermont Quarterly*, Winter 1999.

Ah yes, some will say, but what about drunk driving? They have a point. While it is possible to debate the numbers, there can be little doubt that the higher drinking age has coincided with a reduction in the number of highway deaths. But has the price been worth paying? The question sounds callous, particularly given the horrors of the individual tragedies that make up the statistics, but all legislation is, in the end, a matter of finding a balance between competing rights, interests, and responsibilities. We could, for example, save lives by denying drivers' licenses to those over 65, but we do not. We understand the trade-off: There is an interest in safer roads, but there is also an interest in allowing older people to retain their independence.

In the case of the drinking age, the balance has shifted too far in one direction, away from individual responsibility and towards government control. Raising the limit may have reduced drunken driving, but the cost in lost freedom has been too high, and, quite possibly, unnecessary: Alcohol-related auto accidents seem to be falling in most age categories. The problem of teen DWI [Driving While Intoxicated] is best dealt with directly, by strengthening the deterrents, rather than obliquely, in the context of a wider attack on "under-age" drinking—an attack that might, in fact, ultimately backfire on those whose interest lies in combating the drunk at the wheel.

An Ineffective Law

For the most striking thing of all about the minimum drinking age of 21 is how unsuccessful it has been. A 19-year-old in search of a drink will not have to hunt for long; just ask "Jenna." Almost impossible to police effectively, our current policy sends a signal to the young that our legal system is capricious, weak, occasionally vindictive, and not to be respected. In the interest of enforcing important laws—such as those against drunk driving—we should do what we can to make sure our young people see the police not as interfering busybodies, but as representatives of a mature, broadly respected moral order, who are prepared to treat them as adults. Those who believe government should be in the message-sending business should pay a little more attention to the message they are really sending, when they ask the police to enforce unenforceable—and frankly indefensible—taboos.

| *"D.A.R.E. has played a key role in the overall national drug prevention strategy."*

Drug Education Programs Reduce Teen Drug Use

Joseph A. Santoro

According to Joseph A. Santoro in the following viewpoint, school-based drug education programs, especially D.A.R.E. (Drug Abuse Resistance Education), teach students to resist drugs. He cites several studies finding that teenagers who had completed D.A.R.E. programs were less likely to abuse drugs than teenagers who had not been involved with D.A.R.E. Santoro maintains that D.A.R.E. is an important tool in America's war on drugs. Santoro is the chief of police in Monrovia, California.

As you read, consider the following questions:
1. Why does the author consider the classroom the most promising frontier in the fight against drugs?
2. What is D.A.R.E.'s mission, as stated by the author?
3. According to Santoro, what is the one thing that D.A.R.E. is not?

In Monrovia, California, we believe the most promising frontier in America's longstanding war on drugs is not overseas, in lands ruled by drug overlords, or on the mean streets of America.

The most promising frontier is in the classroom. Classrooms where school children are receiving face-to-face instruction that is giving them the skills and techniques necessary to protect themselves from drug abuse. There is solid truth in the old saying that "an ounce of prevention is worth a pound of cure."

D.A.R.E. (Drug Abuse Resistance Education), with the support of parents and the community, can help reduce the number of children who fall prey to smoking, drinking and illicit drugs. D.A.R.E. is the single largest and most widely used substance abuse prevention program in the world. It is working in Monrovia, and in all 50 states and 54 countries around the world—benefiting over 36 million school children each year.

A 1999 study of 3,150 high school juniors in Ohio found that students who completed two or more semesters of D.A.R.E. in elementary school were 50 percent less likely to become high-risk abusers of drugs and alcohol than were students who were not exposed to D.A.R.E.

The study further concluded that D.A.R.E. strengthens peer resistance skills that enable youths to reject pressures to experiment with drugs or alcohol and students are more likely to discuss with their parents the dangers of getting drunk or using drugs.

Also, a 2000 study of Houston, Texas, schools revealed that students from both middle and high school programs reported a heightened awareness of tobacco, alcohol, drug, weapon, and theft problems on their campus as a result of the D.A.R.E. program. The average response by parents to "Should the D.A.R.E. program be continued?" was 5.85 out of 6. [Thus, the majority of parents wished the program to continue.]

D.A.R.E.'s Mission

D.A.R.E.'s mission is to teach children about the dangers of drugs and provide them with the skills to not just say no—but how to say no. The D.A.R.E. curriculum is periodically revised and enhanced to address the ever-changing needs of young people. But its methods remain the same—don't just lecture kids by saying "drugs are bad"—provide them with credible instructors and the tools to understand and resist the pressures that lead to drugs, alcohol, violence and gangs. By getting the message from a street-wise police officer—one who has been out there—one who knows how drugs and alcohol can destroy lives—kids take that message seriously.

In an effort to continually improve their program, D.A.R.E. has joined forces with the University of Akron and the prestigious Robert Wood Johnson (RWJ) Foundation to evaluate and develop new curricula. D.A.R.E.'s intent is to design the next generation of research-based school curricula for substance abuse and violence prevention. RWJ and the University of Akron have chosen D.A.R.E. as the model to collectively create and maintain the gold standard of drug prevention. Other programs were considered, but D.A.R.E. offered the most potential for addressing the needs of America's youth. The Monrovia Police Department and Monrovia School District are excited to have been selected to participate in a five-year study to help develop a cutting-edge revision of the D.A.R.E. program.

The D.A.R.E. curriculum in Monrovia is taught the way it was designed to be taught. First, we teach basic D.A.R.E. in our fifth grade elementary school classes. It is then reinforced in our seventh grade classes, and later in ninth grade classes. Monrovia officers also teach the D.A.R.E. Parenting Program. This program is held one night per week for six weeks. The Police Department provides free childcare for parents during the classes.

It is well understood by experts that school-based drug prevention must be a part of an overall strategy and reinforcement, which must include continuous drug education, strong community commitment, and most important—parental involvement.

No Magic Wand

Despite all the things that D.A.R.E. is—there is one thing that D.A.R.E. is not—it is not a "magic wand" that will make the

The Effectiveness of D.A.R.E.

Recent studies from Louisiana, Minnesota, and Oregon all have a common message, D.A.R.E. works!

• Released August 20, 2001, The Louisiana D.A.R.E. Evaluation Project surveyed 4,502 students from 40 schools. The evaluation included representation across all racial and economic groups, as well as urban, suburban, and rural schools. Staff surveyed 9th graders to study outcomes of Louisiana's D.A.R.E. programs. The survey was to determine differences between students who had received and those who had not. According to Project's author, Dr. Landry, "D.A.R.E. participants reported significantly lower rates of drug use, use of paraphernalia, binge behavior, and use of readily available over-the-counter drugs."

• Conducted by the University of Minnesota and released in late 2000, The First Minnesota D.A.R.E. Plus School Report was an evaluation of 7th graders to measure their attitudes, behaviors, and beliefs regarding alcohol, tobacco, other drug use and violence. Students in the D.A.RE. program had a statistically significantly lower rate of using alcohol.

• The North Marion, Oregon, D.A.R.E. Research Project was developed to assess the effectiveness of the D.A.R.E. in rural and small towns. Comparison of drug use rates of the 9th grade control group with drug use rates of 8th graders revealed significantly higher rates among the non-D.A.R.E. control group.

Why is it so important to D.A.R.E. to have the best possible program? The answer is simple—the children. Unfortunately, there is no silver bullet to protect America's youth. Any plan must begin with parents and include schools, police, and other components of the community. With a comprehensive K-12 program, as well as a parent program, D.A.R.E. can serve as a foundation from which to build a community shield against the scourge of illegal drugs. Unfortunately, most communities only choose to implement the elementary [program] in reducing drug use.

DARELine International Magazine, Fall 2002.

drug problem in Monrovia, America or anywhere in the world disappear. D.A.R.E. is not and never was intended to be a cure-all to this nation's drug problem—it is, however, an important foundation on which to build drug prevention efforts.

The results of the National Household Survey on Drug Abuse for 2000 show that progress has been made in a key age group, 12–13 year-olds, and that overall drug usage rates have remained stable since the 1999 survey. This annual survey is a highly respected benchmark of illegal drug use in America. It is time to set the record straight—D.A.R.E. has played a key role in the overall national drug prevention strategy that has helped enable America to reach this important milestone.

Community efforts have also played a key role, as has the vital role of individual parents and family members who each day, at home and at work, make this subject one of their highest priorities. The common denominator in the collective efforts of the team—government, law enforcement, health care providers, religious organizations, schools and families—is education. And, although there are many worthwhile prevention programs, none has successfully touched more young people in America than D.A.R.E.

Because of the dedication of the people of D.A.R.E. America, who are never satisfied with the status quo—D.A.R.E. is simply light years ahead of any other drug prevention program—and it is getting better and better every day, one child at a time.

> "*DARE has never been proven to have any lasting effect on the likeliness of children to use drugs later in life.*"

Drug Education Programs Do Not Reduce Teen Drug Use

Ryan H. Sager

In the following viewpoint, *National Review* contributor Ryan H. Sager argues that drug education programs have not had a measurable impact on teen drug use. Citing from research reports and surveys, Sager contends that teenagers who complete D.A.R.E. (Drug Abuse Resistance Education) programs are as likely to experiment with drugs as teenagers who are not exposed to D.A.R.E. He maintains that drug education programs, which often use scare tactics to deter teens from taking drugs, may have the unfortunate consequence of making teens more cynical about anti-substance abuse messages.

As you read, consider the following questions:
1. According to the author, how do D.A.R.E. officials respond to studies that challenge the effectiveness of the program?
2. Why is Joel Brown skeptical of the "no use" approach used by D.A.R.E.?
3. Whose responsibility is it to give teens realistic advice about drugs, in the author's opinion?

Ryan H. Sager, "Teach Them Well: Drug Talk That Fails," *National Review*, vol. 52, May 1, 2000. Copyright © 2000 by National Review, Inc., 215 Lexington Avenue, New York, NY 10016. Reproduced by permission.

Visit a college party, and you're likely to see people smoking cigarettes, drinking alcohol—and quite often, smoking pot and using various other drugs. This scene will horrify some, but it won't surprise anyone familiar with today's college-age youth. Even though the generation of students now in college is the first to have been exposed to anti-drug messages since birth, a large portion of them seem not to have been convinced. By age 18, about 55 percent of students have tried some illicit drug, and 26 percent of college-age kids report having used an illicit drug within the last month. These numbers are up significantly from the beginning of the 1990s. This drug use may or may not represent a serious problem—most of these people go on to lead decent, productive lives—but it does testify to the ineffectiveness of anti-drug education and advertising in this country.

An Expensive Placebo

At a time when educators and the federal government are as committed as ever to the public-private Drug Abuse Resistance Education (DARE) program, and to a new $1-billion five-year taxpayer-funded anti-drug advertising campaign, it is appropriate to evaluate the return we're getting on this investment. If you ask anti-drug activists, some will say these programs have had a demonstrable impact on young people's attitudes toward drugs as well as their use of drugs. Others, however, are concerned that these programs have not proven their worth and could be diverting resources from more effective ways of preventing drug use by young people. According to this view, the public-education front of the drug war has been little more than an expensive placebo.

DARE, which costs approximately $220 million a year (including $1.75 million in taxpayer funding), is by far the most popular anti-drug program in American schools. About 75 percent of school districts use it. While parents and politicians tend to view DARE as sacred, most people are unaware that the program has long faced intense skepticism from experts. Although some studies have found positive effects (mostly attitude changes) over the short term, DARE has never been proven to have any lasting effect on the likeliness of children to use drugs later in life. Numerous studies, in fact, have found that the program has no long-term effect whatsoever. Sending police officers into classrooms to lecture children on the dangers of drugs—the gist of DARE's approach—may lower their opinions of drugs temporarily, but the lessons seem to fade quickly.

For years, DARE officials confronted with these negative studies have dismissed the studies as inadequate in scope. But a recent study by researchers at the University of Kentucky should put those objections to rest. The study examined a group of young people ten years after they completed the DARE curriculum—and concluded that these students were just as likely to use drugs as a group of students who had been exposed to just a minimal drug-education curriculum in their health classes. Though DARE officials have complained that the study should have compared DARE students to students who had received no drug education at all, such a sample would be nearly impossible to find. Furthermore, the argument that DARE should be preserved even if it is no more effective than a shorter and less expensive program seems untenable.

Dissenting Opinions

Charlie Parsons, executive director of DARE America, doesn't believe the University of Kentucky study. He claims the program's curriculum has changed significantly since the period when the tracked students had it, and he puts his own spin on the data: "The effects dissipate somewhat, and that's not a surprise. It shows there's a need for reinforcement, and we totally agree with that." He even offers a solution to any problem that may exist: Extend the DARE program. The students in the University of Kentucky study were exposed to DARE only in elementary school. Mr. Parsons points to a study from Ohio University that shows lower drug use among students who continue with DARE during middle school and high school.

Despite Parsons's optimism, some researchers remain skeptical. Joel Brown, executive director of the Center for Educational Research and Development in Berkeley, questions the validity of the Ohio study on methodological grounds. He also notes that there is still no research show-

Ignoring Reality

Why do people find it so easy to ignore DARE's failure?

The most likely answer is that, in this era of applying touchy-feely solutions to our social problems, DARE is another "feel-good" program. The way people "feel" about it shields it from rational criticism.

The police instructors feel good; they believe that the work they are doing is important. Parents feel good; they believe that something is being done to protect their children from the menace of drug abuse. School officials feel good; they are confident that they are providing the best available program to address the concerns. And politicians feel good; they can project the image of being caring and benevolent.

Such people take satisfaction in the thought that any boy or girl who does not get entangled in drugs has been saved because of the program. They remain oblivious to the reality that the vast majority of these children, even without it, would not have ended up abusing drugs. And they fail to realize that those at risk are unlikely to have been affected by any simplistic, cookie-cutter approach to drug prevention. As one Albertan [from Alberta, Canada] with whom I spoke recently put it: "The kids who were never going to get into drugs anyway thought it was good and those who were going to abuse drugs just did what they were going to do anyway."

If "feel-good" programs like DARE were stopped, we'd likely see no change on the youth drug scene but we would have more time and money to spend on our kids: money to buy necessary school supplies, time to teach necessary skills, and resources to provide effective services to the kids who don't say "no" to drugs.

Tana Dineen, *Report*, February 19, 2001.

ing that the program has any lasting effect.

More generally, Brown is skeptical of the "no-use" approach used by DARE and other programs. "The reality is that most kids will experiment with drugs," he says. He doesn't condone experimentation, but thinks a wiser approach would be "telling kids the truth about drugs trusting young people's ability to make decisions if given information." Brown thinks that kids who are at risk, or who already have problems with drugs, are unable to get useful advice from a program like DARE and could end up in deep trouble. Furthermore, Brown fears that when young people experiment with drugs (or observe others doing so) and find that the dire warnings they heard in DARE were overblown, they will feel that their elders have been lying to them for years. This, he says, could create "cognitive dissonance" that will lead them to reject not just the message but the messenger.

Lacking Balance

The new anti-drug advertising campaign has the same problem: It has little room for a balanced view of drugs and is, for the most part, a variation on the theme of "Just say no." "It's just trying to scare people into not using drugs," says Brown. "There's no evidence that it really has an impact."

Whether or not it has an impact, of course, is an important question, now that the federal government has embarked on a $1-billion ad campaign. But it is almost impossible to study the effects of such a nationwide campaign on kids, because there is no control group—no similar kids who have not seen the ads—to use for comparison.

The Partnership for a Drug-Free America, the organization responsible for most of the anti-drug advertising on television, admits as much. Steve Dnistrian, a Partnership official, points to a correlation between anti-drug advertising and teenage drug use that he believes proves the effectiveness of the new ad campaign. "We're about two years into a very encouraging flattening, if not decline" in teenage drug use, he claims. In fact, according to the University of Michigan's annual Monitoring the Future study, from 1998 to 1999—the study's first opportunity to measure the effect of the new anti-drug ads—teen drug use actually increased (though to a lesser extent than in most years during the 1990s). More important, the flattening to which Dnistrian refers clearly predates the advertising campaign.

A Bleak Picture

What is left after a careful examination of anti-drug education and advertising is a fairly bleak picture for the anti-drug forces. The most widely used drug-education program in America has never proven that it can prevent young people from using drugs, and evidence for the effectiveness of anti-drug advertising is circumstantial at best. Hundreds of millions of dollars go into these programs every year, yet no one can point to any concrete results.

The problem is an anti-drug establishment with no interest in reconsidering its message, or even how the message is delivered. Kids know that smoking one joint will not ruin their lives, so telling them that it will can only make them more cynical than they already are. What we need is a fundamental rethinking of how we talk to kids about drugs. The government is not likely to do this anytime soon—so in the short term, it will be up to parents, alone, to give their kids realistic advice on drugs.

"A 10% increase in the price of cigarettes would lead to a decline of 12% in the number of teenagers who would otherwise smoke."

Higher Cigarette Taxes Would Discourage Teen Smoking

Michael Grossman and Frank J. Chaloupka

In the following viewpoint, Michael Grossman and Frank J. Chaloupka argue in favor of a bill, known as the Hatch-Kennedy Bill after its creators, Senators Orrin G. Hatch and Edward M. Kennedy, that would increase the tax on cigarettes. They contend that increased taxes on cigarettes would reduce teen smoking because teens have little disposable income and would be forced to buy fewer cigarettes as price increased. Moreover, according to the authors, few teenage smokers are addicted to nicotine and thus are unlikely to feel compelled to buy cigarettes as they increase in price. Grossman is a professor of economics at the City University of New York Graduate School. Chaloupka is an associate professor of economics at the University of Illinois at Chicago.

Editor's Note: The Hatch-Kennedy Bill was defeated in 1997.

As you read, consider the following questions:
1. According to the authors, what are three reasons why teenagers are more responsive to cigarette price increases than adults?
2. Why does the effect of a cigarette tax increase grow over time, according to Grossman and Chaloupka?

Numerous studies have shown that roughly 90% of smokers begin the habit as teenagers. Each day, approximately 6000 youths try a cigarette for the first time, and about half of them become daily smokers. Among people who have ever smoked daily, 82% began smoking before age 18. Thus, cigarette control policies that discourage smoking by teenagers may be the most effective way of achieving long-run reductions in smoking in all segments of the population.

The upward trend in teenage smoking in the 1990s is alarming to public health advocates. Between 1993 and 1996 the number of high school seniors who smoke grew by 14%. At the same time the number of tenth grade smokers rose by 23%, and the number of eighth grade smokers rose by 26%. . . .

Legislative Efforts to Reduce Teen Smoking

A 43-cent tax hike is proposed in a bill introduced by Senators Orrin G. Hatch and Edward M. Kennedy in this Congress [as a way of approaching the problem of teen smoking]. As with past tax increases, the primary focus is not to discourage teenage smoking. The goal of the tax increase in the Hatch-Kennedy Bill is to finance health insurance for low-income children who are currently uninsured. Two-thirds of the estimated annual $6 billion increase in tax revenue would be allocated for grants to the states to provide health insurance for children below the age of 18 whose low-income working parents do not qualify for Medicaid. The remaining one-third would be applied to reducing the Federal deficit.

The tobacco industry has known and public health advocates have come to realize, however, that an increase in the cigarette tax can influence the behavior of smokers. The American Cancer Society, the Robert Wood Johnson Foundation, and other members of the antismoking lobby are supporting a proposal to raise state cigarette tax rates to a uniform $2 per pack nationwide in the next few years, from the [1997] range of 2.5 cents in Virginia to 82.5 cents in Washington State. According to John D. Giglio, manager of tobacco control advocacy for the American Cancer Society: "Raising tobacco taxes is our number one strategy to damage the tobacco industry. The . . . industry has found ways around everything else we have done, but they can't repeal the laws of economics."

The cigarette industry's recognition of the potency of excise tax hikes as a tool to discourage teenage smoking is reflected in a September 1981 Philip Morris internal memorandum written by Myron Johnson, a company economist, to his boss, Harry G. Daniel, manager of research on smoking by teenagers. The memo was written in reaction to a National Bureau of Economic Research (NBER) report authored by researchers Michael Grossman, Eugene M. Lewit, and Douglas Coate, which was later published in the *Journal of Law Economics*. In the memo Johnson wrote: "Because of the quality of the work, the prestige (and objectivity) of the NBER, and the fact that the excise tax on cigarettes has not changed in nearly 30 years we need to take seriously their statement that '. . . if future reductions in youth smoking are desired, an increase in the Federal excise tax is a potent policy to accomplish this goal.' [Grossman et al.] calculate that . . . a 10% increase in the price of cigarettes would lead to a decline of 12% in the number of teenagers who would otherwise smoke."

Why Taxes Work

There are strong logical reasons for expecting teenagers to be more responsive to the price of cigarettes than adults. First, the proportion of disposable income that a youthful smoker spends on cigarettes is likely to exceed the corresponding proportion of an adult smoker's income. Second, peer pressure effects are much more important in the case of youth smoking than in the case of adult smoking. Interestingly, peer pressure has a positive multiplying effect when applied to teenage smokers: a rise in price curtails youth consumption directly and then again indirectly through its impact on peer consumption (if fewer teenagers are smoking, fewer other teenagers will want to emulate them). Third, young people have a greater tendency than adults to discount the future.

The "full" price to an individual of a harmful smoking addiction is the price of cigarettes plus the monetary and emotional costs to the individual of future adverse health effects.

The importance and value placed on these future health effects varies among individuals and especially with age. Becker, Grossman, and Murphy have shown that young people are more responsive to the price of cigarettes than adults because they give little weight to the future, while adults are more sensitive to perceived or known future consequences. Young people may underestimate the health hazards of and the likelihood that initiation of this behavior leads to long-term dependency. And, even when fully informed, teenagers have a tendency to give a great deal of weight to present satisfaction and very little weight to the future consequences of their actions. . . .

Estimating Harm

Consumers are not unaware of the dangers of smoking. A survey by researcher W.K. Viscusi suggests that both smokers and nonsmokers overestimate, not underestimate, the probability of death and illness from lung cancer due to tobacco. Teenagers, who have less information than adults, actually attach much higher risks to smoking than the rest of the population. Other risks of cigarette smoking, including the risk of becoming addicted, may, however, be underestimated.

Cigarette smokers harm others (external costs) in addition to harming themselves (internal costs). The ignored internal costs of smoking can interact with the external costs. A striking example is smoking by pregnant teenage women, who may engage in this behavior because they heavily discount the future consequences of their current actions. Pregnant women who smoke impose large external costs on their fetuses. Numerous studies show that these women are more likely to miscarry and to give birth to low birth weight infants. Some of these infants die within the first month of life. More require extensive neonatal intensive care and suffer long-term impairments to physical and intellectual development.

The conventional wisdom argues that people who are addicted to nicotine are less sensitive to price than others. Therefore, adults should be less responsive to price than young people because adult smokers are more likely to be addicted to nicotine and, if so, are likely to be more heavily addicted or to have been addicted for longer periods of time.

Expert Conclusions on Cigarette Prices and Smoking Levels

- The 2000 U.S. Surgeon General's Report, *Reducing Tobacco Use*, found that increasing the price of tobacco products would decrease the prevalence of tobacco use, particularly among kids and young adults, and that tobacco tax increases would lead to "substantial long-term improvements in health." From its review of existing research, the report concluded that raising tobacco taxes is one of the most effective tobacco prevention and control strategies.

- The 1999 World Bank report *Curbing The Tobacco Epidemic: Governments and the Economics of Tobacco Control* carefully evaluated existing research and data, worldwide, and concluded that "the most effective way to deter children from taking up smoking is to increase taxes on tobacco. High prices prevent some children and adolescents from starting and encourage those who already smoke to reduce their consumption."

- Wall Street tobacco industry analysts have long recognized the powerful role increased cigarette taxes and rising cigarette prices play in reducing U.S. smoking levels. For example, a December 1998 "Sensitivity Analysis on Cigarette Price Elasticity" by Credit Suisse First Boston Corporation settled on a "conservative" estimate that cigarette consumption will decline by four percent for every 10 percent increase in price.

- In its 1998 report, *Taking Action to Reduce Tobacco Use*, the National Academy of Sciences' Institute of Medicine concluded that "the single most direct and reliable method for reducing consumption is to increase the price of tobacco products, thus encouraging the cessation and reducing the level of initiation of tobacco use."

- A National Cancer Institute Expert Panel reported in 1993 that "a substantial increase in tobacco excise taxes may be the single most effective measure for decreasing tobacco consumption," and "an excise tax reduces consumption by children and teenagers at least as much as it reduces consumption by adults."

Campaign for Tobacco-Free Kids, "Raising Cigarette Taxes Reduces Smoking, Especially Among Kids (and the Cigarette Companies Know It)," January 3, 2002.

The conventional wisdom that addicted smokers are less sensitive to price has been challenged in a formal economic model of addictive behavior developed by G.S. Becker and

K.M. Murphy, which shows that a price increase can have a cumulative effect over time.

Since cigarettes are addictive, current consumption depends on past consumption. A current price increase has no retroactive effect on "past consumption" and therefore reduces the amount smoked by an addicted smoker by a very small amount in the short run. But the size of the effect would grow over time because even a small reduction in smoking during the first year after a price increase would also mean a reduction in smoking in all subsequent years. So, for example, 10 years after a price hike, "past consumption" would have varied over a 10-year period.

Changes in the total number of young people who smoke are due primarily to changes in the number of new smokers (starts). Among adults, changes in the total number of smokers occur primarily because current smokers quit (quits). Clearly, quits are inversely related to past consumption—there are more quitters among those who have smoked the least—while starts are independent of past consumption. Thus, the effect of price on choosing whether to smoke should be larger for young people than for adults.

The Evidence

Suggestive evidence of the responsiveness of teenage smoking to the price of cigarettes can be found in recent upward trends in smoking. In April 1993, the Philip Morris Companies cut the price of Marlboro cigarettes by 40 cents. Competitors followed suit. Marlboros are popular among teenagers: 60% reported that Marlboro was their brand of choice in 1993, while Marlboro had an overall market share of 23.5% in the same year. In 1993, 23.5% of teenagers in the eighth, tenth, and twelfth grades smoked. In 1996, 28.0% of the students in these grades smoked; this represented a 19% increase over a three-year period. Yet during this period, the number of smokers ages 18 years and older remained the same. Some attribute this increase in teenage smoking to a broad range of social forces thought to be associated with increases in other risky behaviors by teenagers, especially the use of marijuana. But we attribute it to a fall in cigarette prices: between 1993 and 1996 the real price of a pack of cigarettes (the cost of a pack of cigarettes in a given year divided by the Consumer Price Index for all goods for that year) fell by 13%. . . .

In our 1996 study, we used data from the 1992, 1993, and 1994 surveys of eighth, tenth, and twelfth grade students conducted by the Institute for Social Research at the University of Michigan as part of the Monitoring the Future Project. Taken together, these three nationally representative samples included approximately 150,000 young people. We found that a 10% increase in price would lower the number of youthful smokers by 7%, a somewhat smaller effect than the 12% projected in the [E.M. Lewit, D. Coate, and M. Grossman] 1981 study. Consumption among smokers, however, would decline by 6%, which is three times larger than the decline projected in the 1981 study. . . .

Price Increases as a Policy Tool

The proposed 43-cent cigarette tax hike in the Hatch-Kennedy Bill would, if fully passed on to consumers, raise the price of a pack of cigarettes by approximately 23%. According to our 1996 study, the number of teenage smokers would fall by approximately 16% and the number of cigarettes consumed by teenage smokers would decline by approximately 14%. Some of these smokers might compensate for a reduction in the number of cigarettes smoked by switching to higher nicotine and tar brands, inhaling more deeply, or reducing idle burn time. These factors, while representing a pubic health concern, are not relevant in evaluating the effect of an excise tax hike on whether an individual chooses to smoke at all.

Since very few smokers begin smoking after the age of 20, these relatively large reductions in the total number of teenage smokers imply that excise tax increases are very effective ways to prevent the onset of a habitual behavior with serious future health consequences. A 16% decline in the number of young smokers associated with a 43-cent tax hike translates into over 2.6 million fewer smokers in the current cohort of 0 to 17-year-olds. Using a common estimate that one in three smokers dies prematurely from smoking-related illnesses, we can calculate that over time a real (adjusted for inflation) 43-

cent tax increase would reduce smoking-related premature deaths in this cohort by over 850,000. And larger tax increases would result in even bigger reductions in the number of young smokers and the number of premature deaths.

A tax hike would continue to discourage smoking for successive generations of young people and would gradually affect the smoking levels of older age groups as the smoking-discouraged cohorts move through the age spectrum. Over a period of several decades, aggregate smoking and its associated detrimental health effects would decline substantially.

The effect of a price or tax hike also grows over time because of the addictive nature of smoking: a small reduction in current cigarette consumption by smokers due to a tax hike would decrease consumption in all future years to follow. Researchers G.S. Becker, M. Grossman, and K.M. Murphy have estimated that each 10% rise in price causes the number of cigarettes consumed by a fixed population (number of smokers multiplied by cigarettes consumed per smoker) to fall by 4% after one year and by as much as 8% after approximately 20 years. . . .

Focusing on Reducing Teen Smoking

We would like to see politicians and public health advocates focus discussions of the appropriate Federal cigarette excise tax rate squarely on the issue of reducing smoking. Both external costs and ignored internal costs justify the adoption of government policies that interfere with private decisions regarding the consumption of cigarettes.

Taxing cigarettes to reduce smoking by teenagers is a rather blunt instrument because it imposes costs on other smokers. But an excise tax hike is a very effective policy with regard to teenagers because they are so sensitive to price. The current Federal excise tax of 24 cents on a pack of cigarettes is worth about half in real terms of the 8-cent tax in effect in 1951. A substantial real tax hike to curb youth smoking should move to the forefront of the antismoking campaign.

> *"You raise taxes on 98 percent of the smokers, who are the adults, in an effort to try to curtail smoking on 2 percent of the smokers, the young people."*

Higher Cigarette Taxes Would Not Discourage Teen Smoking

John Ashcroft

In the following viewpoint, John Ashcroft argues against passing the 1998 National Tobacco Policy and Youth Smoking Reduction Act, which called for raising federal excise taxes on cigarettes to $1.50 per pack. He contends that the bill targets poor families who constitute the majority of smokers. Ashcroft argues that it is unfair to raise the price of cigarettes just to target teens, who only comprise 2 percent of all smokers. U.S. Attorney General John Ashcroft was a senator from Missouri when this testimony was given.

Editor's note: The Youth Smoking Reduction Act was defeated in 1998.

As you read, consider the following questions:
1. How are communities in Springfield, Missouri, fighting the teen smoking problem, as reported by Ashcroft?
2. According to the author, what steps should Congress take to reduce teen smoking?
3. What is an inevitable outcome of raising taxes on cigarettes, as stated by Ashcroft?

John Ashcroft, testimony before the U.S. Senate, May 20, 1998.

While I will begin my remarks discussing my pending amendment to strike all of the consumer taxes out of the National Tobacco Policy and Youth Smoking Reduction Act, I also wish to address the large expansion of Government in the pending legislation. I will discuss the inevitable black market that will result from the policies in this bill. I will also address the failure of this administration to focus its priorities and resources on teen drug use.

I am truly concerned about teen smoking. However, I do not believe that is the focus of this legislation. Teen smoking is not the central thrust of what is happening here.

Hurting Families

This is a massive, massive tax increase on low-income Americans. Instead of helping children, it is very likely to end up hurting children and hurting families. I think it is important that we carefully review the content of this legislation with that in mind. Thirty-nine percent of high school students in Missouri reported smoking in May 1998. This is a terrible statistic to have to cite. However, communities in the State are looking for ways to reduce smoking in my State and it is working. It is working without destroying the capacity of low-income families to provide for their children. It is working without destroying the capacity of low-income families to be independent. It is working without an $800, or $900, or $1,000, or $1,600 tax increase on those low-income families. Three packs a day for a family at $1.50 a pack takes you to about $1,600 a year.

If we can find a way to reduce the impact of teen smoking without taking $1,600 a year out of the budgets of these poor families, that will be $1,600 a year that could be spent for education, $1,600 a year these families will be able to retain and spend for better health care, or it will be $1,600 a year these families can spend for food and clothing.

For example, I come from a town called Springfield, Missouri. It is my hometown. My family moved there when I was a very young lad. In stepping up its enforcement of local ordinances prohibiting the sale of tobacco products to teens, they are enacting constitutional limitations on advertising. Parents, teachers, and community leaders are working together to fight the problem. They think they can do it, if they work together. I believe they can do it. They can do it without ruining finances and the opportunity that low-income families ought to have to provide for themselves. The tobacco industry knows they can do it. As one tobacco executive stated, they can't win fighting teen smoking rules on the State and local level. The tobacco industry knows there are going to be rules there, and they can be there, and there can be effective rules.

If this tobacco bill contained the solutions to the problems that are being enacted in communities today, I don't think I could be here to argue nearly as effectively that this bill is not focused on teen smoking.

Teen Possession of Tobacco

A lot of communities are making possession of tobacco products illegal for teens. This bill doesn't do that. This bill says it is all right for teens to have tobacco. This bill basically says it is all right for teens to smoke. This bill just says it is wrong to sell it to them and it is wrong to advertise it. But it doesn't really do anything about the possession of tobacco.

Although Congress has the authority, we do not make it illegal for minors to possess or use tobacco even where we control the local situation. We make the laws. We are the city government in some respects for the District of Columbia. It would be possible for us to say, at least where we have authority on military bases, or the District of Columbia, that we could have laws against teen smoking and against the possession of tobacco. But we don't have that in this bill. We only have rules regarding the point of sale. Whether one store or another can sell it, and whether or not they can be on top of the counter or under the counter, or whether or not the brand name can be visible, or things like that, even then we only make the retailers responsible for the transaction. There is no disincentive for teenagers to try to possess and acquire and smoke cigarettes. There is not any in this bill. This is designed as if teenagers are totally expected to be irresponsible. First of all, the decision is, they can't make good decisions; and, second, we don't ask them to make any good decisions. We don't even ask them to refrain from smoking in this bill.

We create a massive tax increase on 98 percent of smokers to try to discourage 2 percent of all retail sales. What do I mean by that? Two percent of all retail sales in smoking go to teenagers; 98 percent go to adults. So we are raising the taxes on 98 percent in order to try to create a disincentive for the 2 percent.

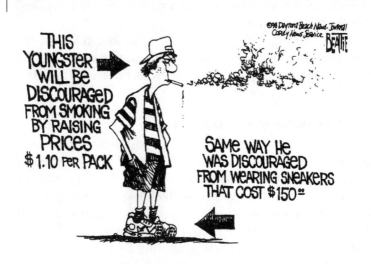

Beattie. © 1998 by *Daytona Beach News Journal*. Reprinted by permission of Copley News Service.

Unfortunately, I don't think we have done a very good job, because we don't even seek to make illegal the possession on the part of the 2 percent. If, in fact, we don't want teenagers smoking, why do we fail to say something about their possession of tobacco? Why do we fail to say anything about their smoking? It seems to me that we are missing the boat in a significant way if we don't say something about the smoking.

Truth in Labeling

For a long time now, we have had a responsibility imposed on the tobacco companies, and appropriately so, to label cigarettes and to tell people the truth about cigarettes on the package. As a matter of fact, you can't even have a billboard about cigarettes without saying on the billboard something that is true about cigarettes. There ought to be said something through this legislation. We need truth in labeling on this legislation. There is a big truth-in-labeling problem here.

This is an $868 billion—that is not million, that is billion—tax increase. It creates Government programs; after-government programs funding, sort of, directed for the next 25 years to take decisionmaking away from future Congresses of the United States, designed to lock things in; creates a huge Government regulatory scheme. . . .

Here you have a situation. You say you are against teen smoking. You don't even bother to outlaw possession of teen tobacco for teens even in places like the District of Columbia where you have the authority to do so. You do not do what lots of towns are doing around the United States of America in an effective program. You raise $868 billion worth of taxes, mostly on poor people, on people who can ill afford to pay it. You raise taxes on 98 percent of the smokers, who are the adults, in an effort to try to curtail smoking on 2 percent of the smokers, the young people.

We create this huge Government regulatory scheme which will have the Federal Government virtually in every store, supermarket, or convenience store telling them how to run their business. This designs a system that will undoubtedly create a black market in tobacco sales, a black market that will make Prohibition look like a very peaceful time in our country's history. Cigarette smuggling will become very, very lucrative. Some people think that smuggling doesn't exist in the United States now. There is a big problem in cigarette smuggling currently, but it is just the tip of the iceberg, which will become apparent if we continue on this plan to impose $1.50 a pack in terms of the cigarette tax on the working poor of America.

Periodical Bibliography

The following articles have been selected to supplement the diverse views presented in this chapter.

Susan Brenna "Eyes Wide Shut," *New York Times Upfront*, September 20, 1999.

Jonathan Chait "The Great Liberal Smokeout: How Democrats Got Hooked on Tobacco Taxes," *New Republic*, May 18, 1998.

George D. Comerci, "Cigarettes, Drugs, Alcohol, and Teens," Paul G. Fuller, and *Patient Care*, February 28, 1997. Sandra F. Morrison

Kris Frieswick "Why Alcohol and Kids Should Mix," *Boston Phoenix*, June 13, 2000.

Stephen Glass "Truth & D.A.R.E.," *Rolling Stone*, March 5, 1998.

D.M. Gorman "The Failure of Drug Education," *Public Interest*, Fall 1997.

Jeffrey J. Hicks "The Strategy Behind Florida's 'Truth' Campaign," *Tobacco Control*, March 2001.

Kathiann M. Kowalski "How Tobacco Ads Target Teens: Tobacco Companies Spend Millions of Dollars on Advertising to Hook More Smokers," *Current Health 2*, April/May 2002.

Mike Males "The Drug Debate Gets Dopier," *AlterNet*, August 20, 2001.

Mike Males and "The Return of Reefer Madness," *Progressive*, Faye Docuyanan May 1996.

Steven C. Manning "Teens & Drugs: How Big a Crisis," *Scholastic Update*, May 2, 1997.

Jacob Sullum "Cowboys, Camels, and Kids: Does Advertising Turn People Into Smokers?" *Reason*, April 1998.

Peter Vilbig "New Highs, New Risks," *New York Times Upfront*, May 8, 2000.

Robert Worth "Making It Uncool," *Washington Monthly*, March 1999.

For Further Discussion

Chapter 1

1. Gene Stephens argues that a variety of factors—such as child abuse, poor health care, and drug abuse—put today's teens at higher risk than teenagers of other generations. Mike Males contends that today's teens are better off than teenagers of other generations; they perform better in school, use fewer drugs, and graduate from college in greater numbers than did their predecessors. Whose evidence do you find most compelling? Explain your answer.

2. According to Peggy O'Mara, Americans' fixation with guns, violence, and consumerism combined with high rates of child abuse and neglect creates angry, violent teenagers. How do the problems she mentions affect your life and the lives of your friends?

3. Kathiann Kowalski contends that peer pressure puts teens at risk of drug or alcohol abuse, smoking, or other dangerous behavior. Have you ever felt pressured to do something you did not want to do? Drawing on your own experience, discuss the role you think peer pressure plays in risk-taking behavior among teens.

4. According to Paula Schleis and Kim Hone-McMahan, gay teenagers suffer physical and verbal abuse from their peers at school. Often, the authors allege, teachers fail to properly punish students who harass gay teens. Do you think that schools should implement more strict punishments for students who abuse their gay classmates? Why or why not?

Chapter 2

1. Robert Rector contends that comprehensive sex education implicitly condones teen sexual behavior by providing students with information about condoms and birth control. Deborah M. Roffman argues that abstinence-only sex education puts teens at risk of becoming pregnant or contracting sexually transmitted diseases. Whose argument do you find most convincing? Explain your answer.

2. According to Dana Mack, teenage parents should be encouraged to marry in order to alleviate the problems of poverty and welfare-dependence commonly associated with teenage childbearing. In Isabel V. Sawhill's opinion, teenage marriages are notoriously unstable and, therefore, are unlikely to create a stable family. Do you think that teenage parents should be encouraged to marry? Citing from the texts, explain why or why not.

3. Kevin Brady argues that federally funded clinics should be required to notify parents before their teenager obtains contraceptives. The Center for Reproductive Law and Policy maintains that reproductive anonymity is a constitutionally protected right. Whose evidence do you find most persuasive? Explain.

Chapter 3

1. Linda J. Collier argues that teenagers who commit violent adult crimes should face adult punishment. Lise A. Young contends that adult punishments are unfair to teenagers because teens are not as cognitively and emotionally mature as adults are. Whose argument do you find most convincing? Examine recent acts of violence committed by teenagers, such as school shootings, and explain why you think the perpetrators should be punished in adult courts or juvenile courts.

2. According to J. Richard Ward Jr., teenage curfew laws reduce the incidence of juvenile crime and protect teenagers from dangerous elements in society. Jordan C. Budd argues that curfew laws do not reduce the incidence of juvenile crime because most youth crime takes place between 3 P.M. and 6 P.M., when curfew laws are not in effect. Drawing on your own experiences, explain why you think curfew laws are effective or ineffective at preventing juvenile crime.

3. Vito A. Gagliardi Jr. contends that zero tolerance laws protect teachers and students from violent crime at school. James Taranto argues that zero tolerance laws unfairly punish students for minor offenses. Whose evidence do you find most compelling and why?

Chapter 4

1. According to Steve Chapman, most teenagers support keeping the minimum drinking age at twenty-one. In your experience, is his assessment correct? Citing from the text, explain why or why not you support keeping the minimum drinking age at twenty-one.

2. Andrew Stuttaford argues that the best way to minimize the problems of teenage alcohol consumption is for parents to teach their teens how to drink responsibly in the home. Do you agree with his argument? Why or why not?

3. Joseph A. Santoro contends that teenagers who are exposed to D.A.R.E. (Drug Abuse Resistance Education) are less likely to abuse drugs than teenagers who are not exposed to D.A.R.E. In Ryan H. Sager's opinion, there is no evidence that D.A.R.E. programs are effective at reducing teen drug use. Did you com-

plete the D.A.R.E. curriculum? Citing from both authors and your own experience, explain whether you think D.A.R.E. is effective and why.

4. According to Michael Grossman and Frank J. Chaloupka, increasing taxes on cigarettes will reduce teen smoking. However, John Ashcroft maintains that raising taxes on cigarettes will unfairly target poor families. With whose argument do you most agree? Explain.

Organizations to Contact

The editors have compiled the following list of organizations concerned with the issues debated in this book. The descriptions are derived from materials provided by the organizations. All have publications or information available for interested readers. The list was compiled on the date of publication of the present volume; the information provided here may change. Be aware that many organizations take several weeks or longer to respond to inquiries, so allow as much time as possible.

Advocates for Youth
1025 Vermont Ave. NW, Suite 200, Washington, DC 20005
(202) 347-5700 • fax: (202) 347-2263
e-mail: info@advocatesforyouth.org
website: www.advocatesforyouth.org

Advocates for Youth believes young people should have access to information and services that help prevent teen pregnancy and the spread of sexually transmitted diseases and enable youth to make healthy decisions about sexuality. The organization publishes brochures, fact sheets, and bibliographies on adolescent pregnancy, adolescent sexuality, and sexuality education.

The Alan Guttmacher Institute
120 Wall St., 21st Fl., New York, NY 10005
(212) 248-1111 • fax: (212) 248-1951
e-mail: info@guttmacher.org • website: www.agi-usa.org

The institute works to protect and expand the reproductive choices of all women and men. It strives to ensure people's access to the information and services they need to exercise their rights and responsibilities concerning sexual activity, reproduction, and family planning. Among the institute's publications are the books *Teenage Pregnancy in Industrialized Countries* and *Today's Adolescents, Tomorrow's Parents: A Portrait of the Americas*, and the report "Sex and America's Teenagers."

American Academy of Child and Adolescent Psychiatry (AACAP)
3615 Wisconsin Ave. NW, Washington, DC 20016
(202) 966-7300 • fax: (202) 966-2891
website: www.aacap.org

AACAP is a nonprofit organization dedicated to providing parents and families with information regarding developmental, behavioral, and mental disorders that affect children and adolescents.

The organization provides national public information through the distribution of the newsletter *Facts for Families* and the monthly *Journal of the American Academy of Child and Adolescent Psychiatry.*

American Civil Liberties Union (ACLU)
125 Broad St., New York, NY 10004
(212) 944-9800 • fax: (212) 869-9065
e-mail: aclu@aclu.org • website: www.aclu.org

The ACLU is a national organization that works to defend Americans' civil rights as guaranteed by the U.S. Constitution. It opposes curfew laws for juveniles and others and seeks to protect the public-assembly rights of gang members or people associated with gangs. The ACLU's numerous publications include the briefing papers "Reproductive Freedom: The Rights of Minors," "Point of View: School Uniforms," and "Equality in Education."

Anorexia Nervosa and Related Eating Disorders, Inc. (ANRED)
PO Box 5102, Eugene, OR 97405
(503) 344-1144
website: www.anred.com

ANRED is a nonprofit organization that provides information about anorexia nervosa, bulimia nervosa, binge eating disorder, compulsive exercising, and other lesser-known food and weight disorders, including details about recovery and prevention. ANRED offers workshops, individual and professional training, as well as local community education. It also produces a monthly newsletter.

Children's Defense Fund (CDF)
25 E St. NW, Washington, DC 20001
(800) CDF-1200 • (202) 628-8787
e-mail: cdfinfo@childrensdefense.org
website: www.childrensdefense.org

The Children's Defense Fund advocates policies and programs to improve the lives of children and teens in America. CDF's Safe Start program works to prevent the spread of violence and guns in schools, and Healthy Start works for universal health care for children. The fund publishes a monthly newsletter, *CDF Reports*, as well as on-line news and reports such as "Children in the States: 1998 Data" and "How to Reduce Teen Violence."

Child Trends, Inc. (CT)
4301 Connecticut Ave. NW, Suite 100, Washington, DC 20008
(202) 362-5580 • fax: (202) 362-5533
e-mail: amoor@childtrends.org • website: www.childtrends.org

CT works to provide accurate statistical and research information regarding children and their families in the United States and to educate the American public on the ways existing social trends— such as the increasing rate of teenage pregnancy—affect children. In addition to the newsletter *Facts at a Glance*, which presents the latest data on teen pregnancy rates for every state, CT also publishes the papers "Next Steps and Best Bets: Approaches to Preventing Adolescent Childbearing" and "Welfare and Adolescent Sex: The Effects of Family History, Benefit Levels, and Community Context."

Drug Policy Alliance
70 W. 36th St., 16th Fl., New York, NY 10018
(212) 613-8020 • fax: (212) 613-8021
e-mail: nyc@drugpolicy.org • website: www.drugpolicy.org

The foundation is dedicated to studying alternatives to the war on drugs. It supports legalization of drug use, though not for minors. It publishes the quarterly *Drug Policy Letter*.

Family Research Council
801 G St. NW, Washington, DC 20001
(202) 393-2100 • fax: (202) 393-2134
e-mail: corrdept@frc.org • website: www.frc.org

The council seeks to promote and protect the interests of the traditional family. It focuses on issues such as parental autonomy and responsibility, community supports for single parents, and adolescent pregnancy. Among the council's numerous publications are the papers "Revolt of the Virgins," "Abstinence: The New Sexual Revolution," and "Abstinence Programs Show Promise in Reducing Sexual Activity and Pregnancy Among Teens."

Family Resource Coalition (FRC)
200 S. Michigan Ave., 16th Fl., Chicago, IL 60604
(312) 341-0900 • fax: (312) 341-9361

The FRC is a national consulting and advocacy organization that seeks to strengthen and empower families and communities so they can foster the optimal development of children, teenagers, and adult family members. The FRC publishes the bimonthly newsletter *Connection*, the report "Family Involvement in Adolescent Pregnancy and Parenting Programs," and the fact sheet "Family Support Programs and Teen Parents."

Focus on the Family
8605 Explorer Dr., Colorado Springs, CO 80920
(719) 531-5181 • fax: (719) 531-3424
website: www.family.org

Focus on the Family is a Christian organization dedicated to preserving and strengthening the traditional family. It believes that the breakdown of the traditional family is in part linked to increases in teen pregnancy, and so it conducts research on the ethics of condom use and the effectiveness of safe-sex education programs in schools. The organization publishes the video *Sex, Lies, and the Truth*, which discusses the issue of teen sexuality and abstinence, as well as *Brio*, a monthly magazine for teenage girls.

Girls, Inc.
30 E. 33rd St., New York, NY 10016-5394
(800) 374-4475 • fax: (212) 683-1253
website: www.girlsinc.org

Girls, Inc. is an organization for girls aged six to eighteen that works to create an environment in which girls can learn and grow to their full potential. It conducts daily programs in career and life planning, health and sexuality, and leadership and communication. Girls, Inc. publishes the newsletter *Girls Ink* six times a year, which provides information of interest to young girls and women, including information on teen pregnancy.

The Heritage Foundation
214 Massachusetts Ave. NE, Washington, DC 20002
(800) 544-4843 • (202) 546-4400 • fax: (202) 546-0904
e-mail: info@heritage.org • website: www.heritage.org

The Heritage Foundation is a public policy research institute that supports the ideas of limited government and the free-market system. It promotes the view that the welfare system has contributed to the problems of illegitimacy and teenage pregnancy. Among the foundation's numerous publications is its Backgrounder series, which includes "Liberal Welfare Programs: What the Data Show on Programs for Teenage Mothers," the paper "Rising Illegitimacy: America's Social Catastrophe," and the bulletin "How Congress Can Protect the Rights of Parents to Raise Their Children."

National Campaign to Prevent Teen Pregnancy
1776 Massachusetts Ave. NW, Suite 200, Washington, DC 20036
(202) 478-8500
website: www.teenpregnancy.org

The goal of the National Campaign to Prevent Teen Pregnancy is to prevent teen pregnancy by supporting values and stimulating actions that are consistent with a pregnancy-free adolescence. The organization publishes the report "Whatever Happened to Childhood? The Problem of Teen Pregnancy in the United States."

The National Center on Addiction and Substance Abuse at Columbia University (CASA)
633 3rd Ave., 19th Fl., New York, NY 10017
(212) 841-5200 • fax: (212) 956-8020
website: www.casa.columbia.org

CASA works to combat all forms of substance abuse and to study the links between substance abuse and other societal problems, including crime, homelessness, and teen pregnancy. The center publishes reports and surveys on the cost, impact, and prevention of substance abuse, including "Substance Abuse and the American Adolescent," "Rethinking Rites of Passage: Substance Abuse on America's Campuses," and the CASA 1997 Back to School Survey, all of which are available on-line.

National Council on Alcoholism and Drug Dependence (NCADD)
20 Exchange Pl., Suite 292, New York, NY 10005
(212) 269-7797 • fax: (212) 269-7510
e-mail: national@ncadd.org • website: www.ncadd.org

In addition to helping individuals overcome addictions, NCADD advises the federal government on drug and alcohol policies and develops substance abuse prevention and education programs for youth. It publishes fact sheets and pamphlets on substance abuse, including the titles *Youth and Alcohol* and *Who's Got the Power? You . . . or Drugs?*

National Institute of Justice (NIJ)
810 Seventh St. NW, Washington, DC 20531
(202) 307-2942 • fax: (202) 307-6394
e-mail: askncjrs@ncjrs.org • website: www.ojp.usdoj.gov

NIJ is the primary federal sponsor of research on crime and its control. It sponsors research efforts through grants and contracts that are carried out by universities, private institutions, and state and local agencies. Its publications include the research briefs

Gang Crime and Law Enforcement Recordkeeping and *Street Gang Crime in Chicago*.

National Institute on Drug Abuse (NIDA)
6001 Executive Blvd., Suite 5213, Bethesda, MD 20892
(301) 443-1125
e-mail: information@lists.nida.nih.gov
website: www.nida.nih.gov

NIDA supports and conducts research on drug abuse—including the yearly Monitoring the Future Survey—in order to improve addiction prevention, treatment, and policy efforts. It publishes the bimonthly *NIDA Notes* newsletter, the periodic *NIDA Capsules* fact sheets, and a catalog of research reports and public education materials, such as "Marijuana: Facts for Teens."

National School Safety Center (NSSC)
141 Duesenberg Dr., Suite 11, Westlake Village, CA 91362
(805) 373-9977 • fax: (805) 373-9277
e-mail: info@nssc1.org • website: www.nssc1.org

NSSC is a research organization that studies school crime and violence, including hate crimes. The center believes that teacher training is an effective means of reducing these problems. Its publications include the book *Gangs in Schools: Breaking Up Is Hard to Do* and the *School Safety Update* newsletter, which is published nine times a year.

Office for Victims of Crime Resource Center
810 Seventh St. NW, Washington, DC 20531
(800) 627-9872
e-mail: askovc@ojp.usdoj.gov • website: www.ojp.usdoj.gov

Established in 1983 by the U.S. Department of Justice's Office for Victims of Crime, the resource center is a primary source of information regarding victim-related issues. It answers questions by using national and regional statistics, research findings, and a network of victim advocates and organizations. The center distributes all Office of Justice Programs publications, including *Female Victims of Violent Crime* and *Sexual Assault: An Overview*.

Office of Juvenile Justice and Delinquency Prevention (OJJDP)
633 Indiana Ave. NW, Washington, DC 20531
(202) 307-5911 • fax: (202) 307-2093
e-mail: askjj@ojp.usdoj.gov • website: ojjdp.ncjrs.org

As the primary federal agency charged with monitoring and improving the juvenile justice system, the OJJDP develops and funds programs on juvenile justice. Among its goals are the prevention and control of illegal drug use and serious crime by juveniles. Through its Juvenile Justice Clearinghouse, the OJJDP distributes fact sheets and reports such as "How Juveniles Get to Criminal Court," "Gang Suppression and Intervention: Community Models," and "Minorities and the Juvenile Justice System."

Partnership for a Drug-Free America
405 Lexington Ave., 16th Fl., New York, NY 10174
(212) 922-1560 • fax: (212) 922-1570
website: www.drugfreeamerica.org

The Partnership for a Drug-Free America is a private, nonprofit coalition of professionals from the communications industry. Based on the belief that changing attitudes is the key to changing behavior, the partnership's mission is to reduce demand for illegal drugs by changing public attitudes about drugs through the media. The partnership's website includes an on-line database of drug information, news about media efforts to stop drug abuse, and other resources for parents and teens.

Sexuality Information and Education Council of the United States (SIECUS)
130 W. 42nd St., Suite 350, New York, NY 10036-7802
(212) 819-9770 • fax: (212) 819-9776
e-mail: SIECUS@siecus.org • website: www.siecus.org

SIECUS develops, collects, and disseminates information on human sexuality. It promotes comprehensive education about sexuality and advocates the right of individuals to make responsible sexual choices. In addition to providing guidelines for sexuality education for kindergarten through twelfth grades, SIECUS publishes the reports "Facing Facts: Sexual Health for America's Adolescents" and "Teens Talk About Sex: Adolescent Sexuality in the 90s" and the fact sheet "Adolescents and Abstinence."

Suicide Awareness\Voices of Education (SA\VE)
PO Box 24507, Minneapolis, MN 55424-0507
(612) 946-7998
e-mail: save@winternet.com • website: www.save.org

SA\VE works to prevent suicide and to help those grieving after the suicide of a loved one. Its members believe that brain diseases such as depression should be detected and treated promptly because they can result in suicide. In addition to pamphlets and the book *Suicide: Survivors—A Guide for Those Left Behind*, the organization publishes the quarterly newsletter *Afterwords*.

Suicide Information and Education Centre
#201 1615 Tenth Ave. SW, Calgary, AB T3C OJ7, CANADA
(403) 245-3900 • fax: (403) 245-0299
e-mail: siec@suicideinfo.ca • website: www.siec.ca/siec.htm

The Suicide Information and Education Centre acquires and distributes information on suicide prevention. It maintains a computerized database, a free mailing list, and a document delivery service. It publishes the quarterly *Current Awareness Bulletin* and the monthly *SIEC Clipping Service*.

Teen STAR Program
Natural Family Planning Center of Washington, D.C.
8514 Bradmoor Dr., Bethesda, MD 20817-3810
(301) 897-9323 • fax: (301) 571-5267
e-mail: hklaus@dgsys.com • website: www2.dgsys.com/~hklaus

Teen STAR (Sexuality Teaching in the context of Adult Responsibility) is geared for early, middle, and late adolescence. Classes are designed to foster understanding of the body and its fertility pattern and to explore the emotional, cognitive, social, and spiritual aspects of human sexuality. Teen STAR publishes a bimonthly newsletter and the paper "Sexual Behavior of Youth: How to Influence It."

Bibliography of Books

Francie M. Berg and Kendra Rosencrans
Children and Teens Afraid to Eat: Helping Youth in Today's Weight-Obsessed World. Hettinger, ND: Healthy Weight Network, 2000.

Neil I. Bernstein
How to Keep Your Teenager Out of Trouble and What to Do If You Can't. New York: Workman, 2001.

William Lee Carter
It Happened to Me: A Teen's Guide to Overcoming Sexual Abuse. Oakland, CA: New Harbinger, 2002.

Gwendolyn Mitchell Diaz
Sticking Up for What Is Right: Answers to the Moral Dilemmas Teenagers Face. Colorado Springs, CO: NavPress 2002.

Sean Donahue
Gangs: Stories of Life and Death from the Streets. New York: Thunder's Mouth, 2002.

David Elkind
All Grown Up and No Place to Go: Teenagers in Crisis. Reading, MA: Addison-Wesley, 1998.

David K. Freman
Running Away. Salt Lake City, UT: Benchmark, 1996.

Maggie Gallagher
The Age of Unwed Mothers: Is Teen Pregnancy the Problem? New York: Institute for American Values, 1999.

Bernard Golden
Healthy Anger: How to Help Children and Teens Manage Their Anger. Oxford, England: Oxford University Press, 2003.

Ted Gottfried
Homelessness: Whose Problem Is It? Brookfield, CT: Millbrook, 1999.

Ted Gottfried
Teen Fathers Today. Breckenridge, CO: Twenty First Century, 2001.

Patricia Hersch
A Tribe Apart: A Journey into the Heart of American Adolescence. New York: Ballantine, 1998.

Lou Holtz and Matt Smith
A Teen's Game Plan for Life. Notre Dame, IN: Sorin, 2002.

Sam Horn
Take the Bully by the Horns: Stop Unethical, Uncooperative, or Unpleasant People from Running and Ruining Your Life. New York: St. Martin's, 2002.

Cheri Huber and June Shiver
There Is Nothing Wrong with You: For Teens. Murphys, CA: Keep It Simple, 2001.

Tracy Hughes
Everything You Need to Know About Teen Pregnancy. New York: Rosen, 1999.

Harold S. Koplewicz
More than Moody: Recognizing and Treating Adolescent Depression. New York: Penguin, 2002.

Christine Wickert Koubeck
Friends, Cliques, and Peer Pressure: Be True to Yourself. Berkeley Heights, NJ: Enslow, 2002.

Nancy Lesko	*Act Your Age! A Cultural Construction of Adolescence.* New York: Routledge, 2001.
Cynthia Lightfoot	*The Culture of Adolescent Risk-Taking.* New York: Guilford, 1997.
Jose M. Lopez	*Gangs: Casualties in an Undeclared War.* Dubuque, IA: Kendall/Hunt, 2002.
Dana Mack	*The Assault on Parenthood: How Our Culture Undermines Parenthood.* San Francisco, CA: Encounter 2000.
Eric Marcus and Jane O'Connor	*What If Someone I Know Is Gay? Answers to Questions About Gay and Lesbian People.* New York: Price Stern Sloan, 2000.
Adam Mastoon	*The Shared Heart: Portraits and Stories Celebrating Lesbian, Gay, and Bisexual Young People.* New York: HarperCollins, 2001.
Richard C. McCorkle and Terrence D. Miethe	*Panic: The Social Construction of the Street Gang Problem.* Upper Saddle River, NJ: Prentice Hall, 2001.
Jeylan T. Mortimer and Reed Larson	*The Changing Adolescent Experience: Societal Trends and the Transition to Adulthood.* New York: Cambridge University Press, 2002.
Lynn E. Ponton	*The Romance of Risk: Why Teenagers Do the Things They Do.* New York: Basic, 1997.
Lynn E. Ponton	*The Sex Lives of Teenagers: Revealing the Secret World of Adolescent Boys and Girls.* San Diego, CA: Dutton/Plume, 2001.
Deborah M. Roffman	*Sex and Sensibility: The Thinking Parent's Guide to Talking Sense About Sex.* Cambridge, MA: Perseus, 2001.
Nancy L. Snyderman and Peg Streep	*Girl in the Mirror: Mothers and Daughters in the Years of Adolescence.* Sunnyvale, CA: Hyperion, 2003.
Laura Sessions Stepp	*Our Last Best Shot: Guiding Our Children Through Early Adolescence.* New York: Riverhead, 2000.
Barbara Strauch	*The Primal Teen: The New Discoveries About the Teenage Brain and How They Explain Teenage Behavior.* New York: Doubleday, 2003.
Margi Trapani	*Listen Up! Teenage Mothers Speak Out.* New York: Rosen, 1997.
Emily White	*Fast Girls: Teenage Tribes and the Myth of the Slut.* New York: Scribner, 2002.
Rosalind Wiseman	*Queen Bees and Wannabes: A Parent's Guide to Helping Your Daughter Survive Cliques, Gossip, Boyfriends, and Other Realities of Adolescence.* New York: Crown, 2002.

Index